Risk Management for Dysphagia:
Application of Hazard & Operability Study (HAZOP)

Editor
Masanaga Yamawaki & Tohru Nomura

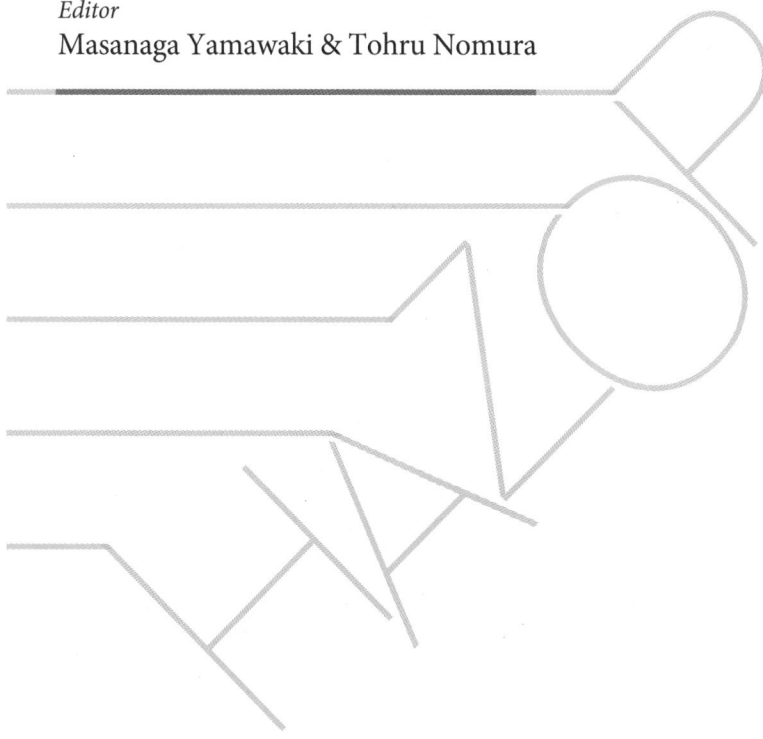

University Education Press

Acknowledgment

"*Most importantly, we must systematically design safety into processes of care.*"

(In "To Err is Human" by WC Richardson)

The basic concept of this book summarizes in the sentence above. The aim of this book is to clarify the aspiration risk by system-based analysis: HAZOP (Hazard and Operability Study). HAZOP can be performed with interdisciplinary healthcare team and be applied in daily clinical settings.

This book was supported by the Grant-in-Aid for Publication of Scientific Research Results of Japan Society for the Promotion of Science (JSPS), #215221.

I gratefully acknowledge the crucial contribution of all the authors: Dr. Tohru Nomura, Dr. Atsushi Okawa, Dr. Mitsuko Shimizu, Dr. Yumi Chiba, and Dr. Haruka Tohara. The preparation of this book greatly benefited from the close scrutiny of Dr. Tohru Nomura for Japanese edition. I would also like to thank the publishers. Their trust and support was very precious. Last but not least, a word of thanks cannot suffice to express my feelings for my wife and my son, who patiently supported me during the long months spent exploring and writing about the universe of dysphagia. This book is dedicated to all of them.

Masanaga Yamawaki
Tokyo, Japan
February 2010

Table of Contents

Acknowledgment ··· *1*

Chapter 1
Risk Management in Swallowing Movement ······················· *9*
  A) Eating and Swallowing   *9*
  B) Dysphagia and Aspiration Pneumonia   *12*
  C) Mechanism of Dysphagia and Risk Management   *16*
  D) Examination for Dysphagia: Evaluation System for Aspiration Risk   *21*
  E) Risk Analysis by HAZOP   *24*

Chapter 2
Medical HAZOP ··· *25*
  A) HAZOP (Hazard and Operability Study)   *25*
  B) Medical HAZOP   *30*

Chapter 3
HAZOP for Swallowing Disorders ···································· *48*

Chapter 4
Application of HAZOP for Risk Management in Dysphagia ············ *54*
  4.1   Medical HAZOP in Clinical Settings ·································· *54*
    A) Challenges for medical accidents   *54*
    B) A model for developing safety management   *63*
    C) Application of medical HAZOP   *67*
  4.2   Risk Communication and HAZOP ···································· *70*
    A) Risk communication using risk matrix   *70*
    B) Category of human factor and HAZOP   *73*
    C) Human factors and guidewords in HAZOP   *77*

4.3　HAZOP and Rehabilitation for Dysphagia ·················· 79
　　A) Swallowing phases and risks　79
　　B) Pharyngeal Phase　80
4.4　Application to Clinical Pathway ························· 92
　　A) Clinical Pathway in health care　92
　　B) Application of HAZOP to Clinical Pathway　96
4.5　Application of HAZOP to In-Home Care ················ 102
　　A) Tips for organizing care team for dysphagia　104
　　B) Case presentation　107
4.6　Application to Basic Research for Dysphagia ············ 110
　　A) Application to basic research for dysphagia　110
　　B) Research on swallowing control　116

List of Tables and Figures

Tables

Table 1.1 Swallowing process and P&ID ... *12*
Table 1.2 Survey of dysphagia in Japan ... *14*
Table 1.3 Five phases of swallowing movement ... *16*
Table 1.4 Mechanism of airway protection ... *20*
Table 1.5 Organs with valve function for swallowing ... *20*
Table 1.6 Definition of HAZOP terminology in dysphagia analysis ... *24*
Table 2.1 Methods for risk assessment and cause/result ... *25*
Table 2.2 An example of WBS ... *27*
Table 2.3 Process Keywords (First Group) ... *28*
Table 2.4 Process Keywords (Second Group) ... *29*
Table 2.5 HAZOP Guidewords ... *29*
Table 2.6 Comparison of Process Safety Management in industry and medicine ... *35*
Table 2.7 Work Breakdown Structure (WBS) Sheet ... *42*
Table 2.8 Basic Guidewords (secondary keywords) ... *44*
Table 2.9 HAZOP Sheet ... *45*
Table 2.10 Level of medical accident/incident in Japan ... *46*
Table 2.11 Classification of frequency ... *46*
Table 3.1 Nodes and subnodes in swallowing process ... *48*
Table 3.2 Deviation in SW4-3 (Laryngeal elevation) ... *50*
Table 3.3 Deviation of Less in SW4-3 (Laryngeal elevation) : analysis of effects and cause ... *50*
Table 3.4 Deviation of Less in SW4-3 (Laryngeal elevation) : analysis of frequency and impact ... *51*
Table 3.5 Analysis of risk rank in each node ... *53*
Table 4.1 Contents and degree of accidents in 2006 (Japan) ... *56*
Table 4.2 Site and degree of accident in 2006 ... *57*
Table 4.3 Risks for falls (brainstorming) ... *69*
Table 4.4 HAZOP guidewords related to human factors ... *78*
Table 4.5 HAZOP for human factors in medication ... *79*
Table 4.6 Progress of Clinical Pathway ... *95*
Table 4.7 Objectives and results of Clinical Pathway ... *96*
Table 4.8 Acute phase: WBS in physical assessment ... *98*

Table 4.9 Time cource of execution ·········· *101*

Table 4.10 Role for management for deglutition disorder ·········· *104*

Table 4.11 WBS of training for dysphagia based on the first examination ·········· *108*

Table 4.12 Tips for team care·········· *110*

Table 4.13 Node ingestion and bolus formation ·········· *112*

Table 4.14 Node from closure of nasopharynx to cough reflex ·········· *114*

Table 4.15 Gvideword and deviation ·········· *117*

Figures

Figure 1.1 Structures involved in swalowing·········· *10*

Figure 1.2 Piping and Instrumentation Diagram (P&ID) in swallowing ·········· *11*

Figure 1.3 Cause of dysphagia (in-home service) ·········· *13*

Figure 1.4 Route of nutrition ·········· *14*

Figure 1.5 Route of tube feeding ·········· *15*

Figure 1.6 Bolus in oral phase Circles are points to produce pressure ·········· *17*

Figure 1.7 Bolus in pharyngeal phase ·········· *18*

Figure 2.1 HAZOP Flow Chart ·········· *31*

Figure 2.2 Frame of risk management (BS31100)·········· *37*

Figure 2.3 Heinrich's law ·········· *43*

Figure 2.4 Objectives and procedure for HAZOP ·········· *44*

Figure 2.5 Risk Matrix ·········· *47*

Figure 3.1 Risk matrix in SW4.3-1 ·········· *52*

Figure 4.1 Factors influencing medical qualiy ·········· *60*

Figure 4.2 Black box of risks ·········· *66*

Figure 4.3 Risks from prescription to injection ·········· *66*

Figure 4.4 Swiss Cheese model ·········· *71*

Figure 4.5 PERT and Clinical Pathway ·········· *93*

Figure 4.6 Flows in Clinical Pathway ·········· *97*

Figure 4.7 Critical Pathway and contents ·········· *99*

Figure 4.8 Clinical Pathway and estimated risk·········· *100*

Figure 4.9 Time course of execution of contens ·········· *101*

Figure 4.10 Team members associated with dysphagia care ·········· *103*

Figure 4.11 Examination of Dysphagia ·········· *105*

Figure 4.12 Two types of team approach ·········· *106*

Figure 4.13 Timeline of the patient with dysphagia ·········· *109*

Figure 4.14 Cerebral control of swallowing movement·········· *111*

Figure 4.15 Sequential movement of deglutition (Jean A. Physiological Rev. 2001.) ········ *111*
Figure 4.16 Theoretical backgrounds of NIRS ·· *118*
Figure 4.17 Localizafion of swallowing component ·· *119*
Figure 4.18 Command Swallow (n=25) ·· *120*
Figure 4.19 Command VS. Non-command (subtracted n=25) ···························· *121*

Risk Management in Swallowing Movement

Chapter 1

A) Eating and Swallowing

There are various meanings of eating for humans other than to take nutrition. For instance, to prevent and treat illness, to express the feeling of love and anxious, to maintain human relations, to unravel a mental and emotional stress, to make others know a social status, to express a faith, and to enjoy a meal purely. The behavior of eating comprise not only as physical or physiological meaning, but mental, social, and cultural meanings. Thus the act of eating includes various values, and disorder of swallowing movements, which is referred to as dysphagia, have much influence on the quality of our life.

Usually, to eat or to drink starts with consciousness for ingestion and swallowing. Moreover, if food goes into throat from mouth, subsequent operation cannot be stopped by will, and it will go to stomach automatically. Drinking liquid or eating food is controlled by the voluntary action (which is possible with one's intention) and the involuntary movement (unconscious with an unrelated intention). The center of this control is located in the brain. The instructions about various swallowing functional operation take place from a cerebrum and the brain stem. These instructions get across to cranial nerves, and move the muscles of tongue and throat. On the other hand, from the sensory receptor of tongue and throat, the sensation of food is continuously sent to the brain.

A swallowing function is classified into five phases functionally and anatomically. That is, the phase to understand and prepare to eat food (recognition phase), the phase when saliva is mixed and food is made to swallow (preparation phase), the phase when food (bolus) press out to throat (oral phase), the phase when bolus pass through pharynx (pharyngeal phase), and the phase when bolus pass to stomach (esophageal phase). Thus, by operation called swallowing, a voluntary action and an involuntary movement cooperate, and bolus goes to the stomach so that food and liquid may flow smoothly.

Abnormalities in any portion of the network, the PC (brain), electric wire (nerve), and a motor (muscles), cause dysphagia. Since neurological diseases, such as cerebral infarction and Parkinson's disease, affect the course from brain to muscles, they cause dysphagia in many cases. Moreover, otolaryngological diseases, gastrointestinal diseases, orthopedic diseases may cause dysphagia. Furthermore, especially in elderly people, even if there is no illness, deglutition disorder may occur. About swallowing disorder caused by these diseases, research of the functional mechanism progresses in recent years, the pattern of an insufficiency is classified, and future prospects (prognosis), medical treatments, and rehabilitation methods are studying.

An important point when considering the risk of dysphagia is a phenomenon of aspiration which food may fall into lung and may cause pneumonia. Since a trachea

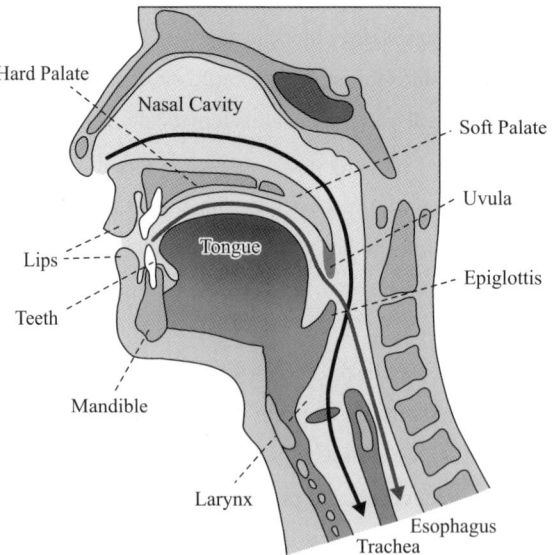

Figure 1.1 Structures involved in swallowing

Chapter 1 Risk Management in Swallowing Movement 11

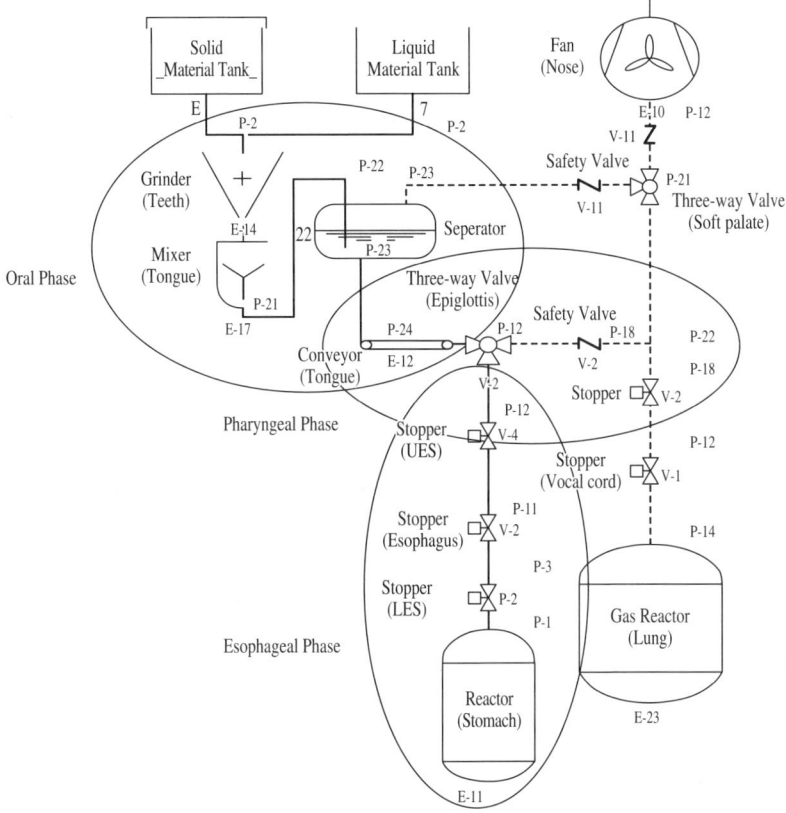

Figure 1.2 Piping and Instrumentation Diagram (P&ID) in swallowing

is a passage of breathing, suffocation and pneumonia are developed by aspiration. This type of pneumonia is called aspiration pneumonia, and has a feature which become seriously ill and chronic. With the disease which causes a swallowing difficulty, aspiration pneumonia determines life prognosis in many cases. Chronic aspiration occurred without obvious symptom (like coughing) is called silent aspiration and becomes frequent with age. In order to avoid the risk of aspiration, it is necessary to control traffic in the passage of air and food correctly in the case of swallowing movement. A swallowing difficulty is generated by the breakdown of this minute control mechanism. Conventionally, although HAZOP analysis was

Table 1.1 Swallowing process and P&ID

	Swallowing Process	Process in Chemical Plant	Receptors
Recognition Phase	Recognization of food and start ingestion	**Material Tank** Receipt and investigation of food	Outlook Checker for volume Analyzer Thermometer
Preparatory Phase	Ingestion and mastication to form bolus	**Grinder and Mixer** Grind and mix of solid and liquid Produce mixture Pore chemical liquid (saliva) to the mixture	Thermometer Sensor for poison Sensor of volume Analyzer of grains Analyzer of texture
Oral Phase	Formation bolus and transfer from oral cavity to pharynx	**Conveyer** Transfer of bolos	Sensor for volume Sensor for conveyer
Pharyngeal Phase	Closure of upper and lower airway and transfer of bolus from pharynx to esophagus	**Seperator** Closure of upper and lower gas pipe Transfer of bolus mixture to solid/liquid pipe through two ducts (priform sinus)	Receptor for closure of gas pipe Receptor for opening for lquid/solid pipe
Esophageal Phase	Phase from entrance of esohagus to stomach	**Conveyer of liquid/solid mixture with two volves**	First volve (entrance volve to esophagus) Sensor for conveyer Second volve (exit volve to stmach)

a technique currently used for the risk assessment of a chemical plant, swallowing movement can be expressed as a chemical plant figure, which is the theme of this book. (Fig 1.1, 1.2, Tab 1.1)

B) Dysphagia and Aspiration Pneumonia
1) Incidence of Dysphagia and Aspiration Pneumonia

Among the patients with cerebrovascular disease it is reported that 22% to 65% of patients suffered from swallowing difficulty. Dysphagia is often associated with aspiration pneumonia, which results in an important factor for the life prognosis and QOL (quality of life) of a patient. Moreover, patients of aspiration pneumonia spend 21 to 40 hospital days, and medical expenses of 9,460 to 33,430 dollars are

Chapter 1 Risk Management in Swallowing Movement 13

estimated in U.S. Thus, the prediction and prevention of aspiration pneumonia is important from the field of medical cost and preventive medicine. However, the exact frequency of the swallowing difficulty and aspiration pneumonia was unknown in any country.

Then, we conducted large-scale investigation for medical institutions all over the country, the welfare institution for elderly people, and the home nursing station about the frequency of dysphagia, aspiration pneumonia, and the nutrition method. We collected the questionnaires of 50,607 examples from 2,867 institutions in total. Main purpose of this survey is 1) the frequency of patients with dysphagia, 2) the frequency of aspiration pneumonia, 3) the frequency of silent aspiration, and 4) nutrition method in patients with dysphagia. As a result, the frequency of patients with dysphagia is 28.5% in nursing home, 17.7% in-home visit, and 14.7% in hospitals (Fig 1.3, Tab 1.2). The frequency of acute aspiration pneumonia is 3.9 to 11.0% , and it is estimated that 1.15% to 1.60% of total patients in facilities suffered from aspiration pneumonia. Moreover, the past history of dysphagia is 56.3% in-home visit, 42.0% in hospitals, and 35.3% in nursing home. 5.6 to 11.7% of patients with aspiration pneumonia did not show signs of coughing or choking, and these patients reveal silent aspiration. About half of dysphagia patients ingest orally, and nutrition route by PEG was mostly used for the patient who cannot carry out oral

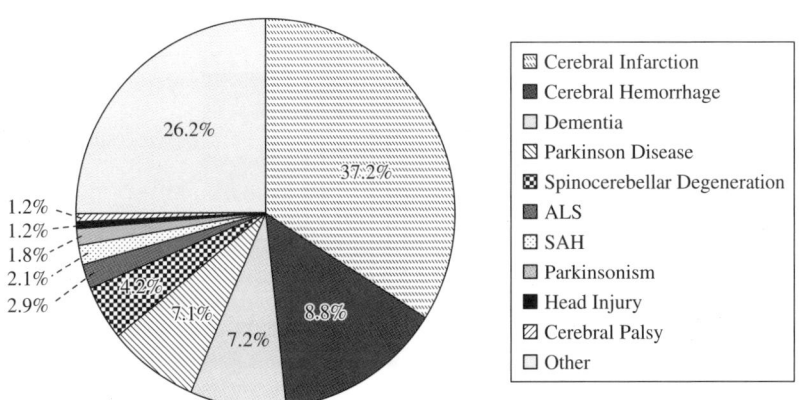

Figure 1.3 Cause of dysphagia (in-home service)

Table 1.2 Survey of dysphagia in Japan

	Hospital	Nursing Home	In-Home Care
Number of facilities	1,053	841	712
Number of all the patients	188,156	43,234	33,374
Number of patients with dysphagia	27,659	12,759	5,907
Dysphagia/All the patients (%)	14.7	29.5	17.7
Aspiration pneumonia (%)	1.60	1.15	1.40
Aspiration pneumonia/Dysphagia (%)	11.0	3.9	7.6
Aspiration pneumonia (past history) (%)	42.0	35.3	56.7
Silent aspiration (%)	11.70	7.63	5.58

ingestion (Fig 1.4, 1.5).

The age composition of the population in Japan increase gradually, and the rate of population aged 65 and over was 17.2% in 2000. It is estimated to reach to 26.9% in 2020 and to 32.3% in 2050. The prevalence rate of the disease which needs care with aging is also increasing. Especially, as a bedridden cause, cerebrovascular diseases forms about 40% of elderly people's bedridden cause, and has become the cause of reducing QOL. Stroke causes swallowing difficulty simultaneously in many cases, and prevention of aspiration and pneumonia becomes an important challenge for the medical person and the care worker.

The evaluation of dysphagia in consideration of disease recovery process is also an important viewpoint. Although the incidence of dysphagia after stroke varies

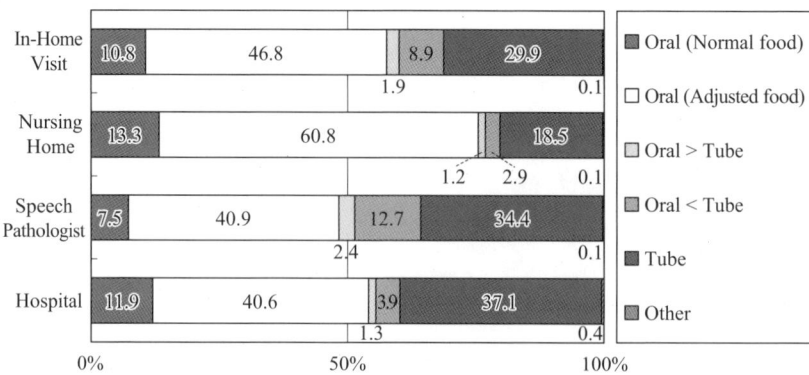

Figure 1.4 Route of nutrition

Chapter 1 Risk Management in Swallowing Movement 15

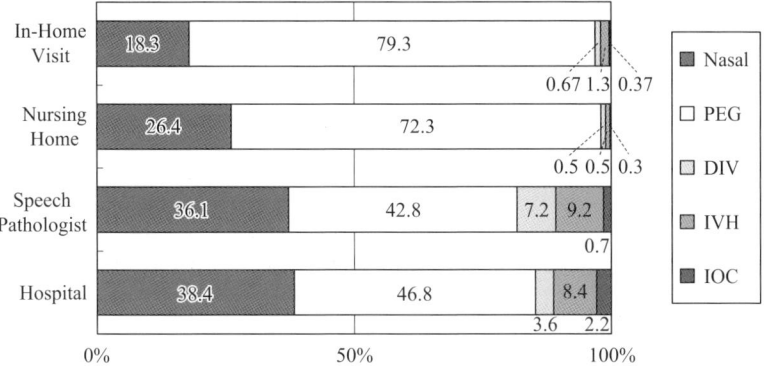

Figure 1.5 Route of tube feeding

according to reports, it is estimated from 22% to 65%. By videofluorographic study (VFSS) dysphagia is reported in 65% of patient with stroke within five days and in 80% within one week. In the acute phase of stroke, 51 to 73% patients with dysphagia result in aspiration, and it is reported that aspiration raises the relative risk of pneumonia 6.95 times. Since it takes into consideration that 34% of stroke patients is dead by pneumonia, the measure against dysphagia and aspiration is important also from the viewpoint not only of the life prognosis and QOL of a patient, but medical-expenses and cost efficiency. After an acute phase, 80% or more of patient with dysphagia is recovered within 2 to 4 weeks. According to the report of Smithard, the prevalence rate of dysphagia is 80% at onset, 27% on the 7th day, 17% after one month, and 11% after six months. In another analysis, incidence of aspiration pneumonia is reported 10.9 % in a week, 0.5 % in four weeks, and 0.2 % in 12 weeks after the onset of stroke. The most important point is the timing when dysphagia patient begin oral ingestion considering the risk of aspiration. In many cases whether oral ingestion is possible for a patient is determined by experience of doctor, nurse, or speech pathologist, and judgment may not be based on the evidence.

As riskfactors of aspiration pneumonia for patients with stroke, mechanical ventilation, multiple brain lesion, verteblobasilar lesion, deglutition disorder, abnormal chest X-rays are reported. Moreover, it is reported to be influenced by a consciousness level and the existence of tube nutrition. In this book our basic investigation is focused on cases who can start oral ingestion in chronic phase of stroke, however, there are many cases who still remains tube feeding because of dysphagia and aspiration.

These data indicate that it is our important mission how correctly we can perform risk assessment and management of dysphagia in the future aging society.

C) Mechanism of Dysphagia and Risk Management
1) Mechanism of Swallowing Movement and Disorders

In HAZOP analysis, the first thing is to perform structured investigation of a movement process (WBS: creation of Work Breakdown Structure, after-mentioned). The process of swallowing movement can actually be expressed in chemical plant, as shown in the figures (Figure 1.1 and 1.2). The process of swallowing movement is classified functionally and anatomically into five phases. That is, the recognition phase in which we are going to understand and eat food, the preparatory phase in which we mix saliva and form bolus, the oral phase in which bolus is sent to the pharynx from the mouth, the pharyngeal phase in which bolus passes pharynx so that it may not go into a trachea, and the esophageal phase which bolus is transferred into stomach (Table 1.3). This process is roughly classified into ingestion (from recognition to preparation phase) and swallowing (from oral to esophageal phase). In ingestion conditions such as cognitive state, tabling, and oral care are involved, and in swallowing involuntary mechanism serves as movement mechanism.

Table 1.3 Five phases of swallowing movement

Recognition phase	Understand food and start ingestion
Preparatory phase	Ingestion and mastication to form bolus
Oral phase	Transfer bolus to pharynx
Pharyngeal phase	Transfer bolus through pharynx
Esophageal phase	Transfer bolus through esophagus

2) Swallowing Process
a) Preparatory Phase
The phase to prepare bolus, and there are three steps, predation, digestion, and the bolus formation.
b) Oral Phase (Figure 1.6)
After bolus is formed, in order to transport it to the pharynx from the mouth, various movements start in 0.5 seconds. Vocal cords are adducted first, operation of tongue and hyoid starts, and lips close. Furthermore, vocal folds are closed and UES opens. Operation of tongue is important in oral phase and makes bolus move. Tongue margin is firmly attached to the hard palate, and bolus is sent in. External tongue muscle is contracted at the moment of swallowing so that bolus may be pushed out backward (to pharynx). A hyoid is elevated by this motion to the front. The rear tongue is carried out by the palatoglossus muscle on elevation. Simultaneously, movement behind tongue makes hyoid kickback on elevation to the position at the angle of mandible, and this elevated position is maintained during swallowing movement. Closing of the nosopharynx is completed by a velar elevation. Moreover, airway obstruction also starts in oral phase simultaneously for laryngeal protection. The blockade of both vocal cords and vocal folds are also important.

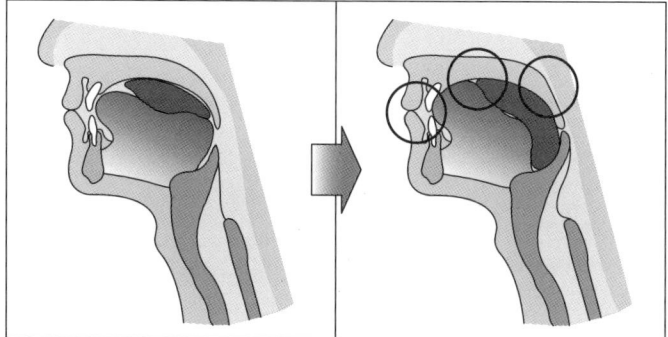

Figure 1.6 Bolus in oral phase
Circles are points to produce pressure.

c) Pharyngeal Phase (Figure 1.7)

Pharyngeal phase is a process where most organs are involved and operated dynamically. Various organs, such as epiglottis, pyriform sinus, hyoid, thyroid and annular cartilage, larynx, and laryngeal wall, move continuously. Pharyngeal muscles will be carried out on elevation and will be shortened when bolus arrives. With movement of thyroid cartilage and annular cartilage, larynx holds on elevation to the front upper part. The epiglottis closes the upper part respiratory tract entrance with laryngeal elevation, and bolus is guided to the esophagus instead of to the respiratory tract. Elevation of larynx (2 to 3cm) produces negative pressure in lower pharynx part. Bolus moves into the pharynx in the portion of epiglottic vallecula from sublingual region, and it avoids going to respiratory tract. The respiratory tract protection mechanism are shown in Table 1.4. The constrictor muscle of pharynx shortens the pharynx narrowly simultaneously, and positive pressure is produced by nose pharynx closing by the velum. The contraction time of this pharyngeal muscle is not based on bolus size. Bolus goes to the superior pyriform sinus of the bottom pharynx, and joins in the UES.

Bolus remaining at tongue base, epiglottic vallecula, and pyriform sinus after the end of a swallowing movement is called pharyngeal residues. It is important at bedside to take medical history of the existence of a feeling of remains in pharynx. When remains are seen in VFSS, we should check the existence of a feeling of residues. Furthermore, it should be confirmed whether these remains disappear by

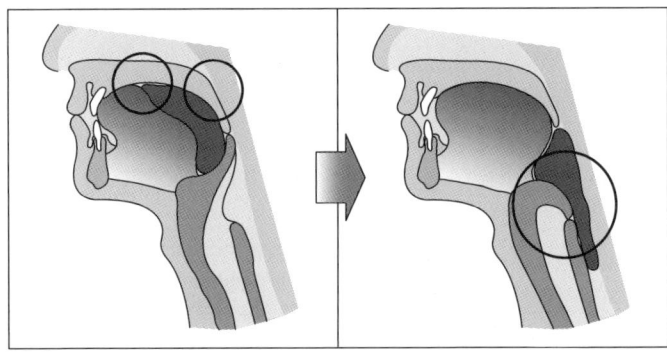

Figure 1.7   Bolus in pharyngeal phase

continuation swallowing. A feeling of residues may be based not only on what is depended on motility disturbance but on decrease of saliva secretion, and it will change with oral condition. When there is much residual volume, a risk of aspiration becomes high.

d) Esophageal Phase

Sympathetic nerve from upper cervical ganglion keeps UES closed except the time of swallowing. The stimulus of parasympathetic system carries out relaxation and opening of the UES at the time of belch, of nausea, and of swallowing. Furthermore, three mechanisms are associated in the opening of UES; UES relaxation accompanying pharynx contraction, mechanical opening by hyoid elevation, positive pressure which pushes out bolus to esophagus. Bolus size regulates the opening mechanism of UES. If bolus is large, nervous activity of UES at the time of swallowing will be activated at an early stage, and opening time will also be prolonged.

When bolus goes into esophagus, a peristalsis is generated from oral side to stomach side. The first wriggle wave is the largest, and the strength of a wriggle is influenced by the residual substance and clearance of pharynx. A wriggle will also become strong if pharyngeal clearance is good. Operation of the same bolus under multiple swallow inhibits a wriggle. The 2nd wriggle wave occurs in relation to spread of bolus in the esophagus. This 2nd wriggle wave sends the signal of LES opening. Although the bolus transfer of an esophagus varies with the texture, it takes 3 to 10 seconds.

3) Critical Points for Swallowing Movement

a) Blockade of Airway (Table 1.4, Table 1.5)

Velum palatinum is raised, and an upper airway is closed by being pushed against the posterior pharyngeal wall. Furthermore, hyoid and larynx elevate with contraction of base of oral cavity, and larynx approaches to epiglottis. Epiglottis is pushed by tongue base and sinks, and laryngeal aperture is closed. Closing of vocal cord and the stop of breathing take place simultaneously. A lower airway is intercepted by the above mechanism.

Table 1.4 Mechanism of airway protection

Lower airway closure	Vocal cord and vocal fold close.
Elevation of larynx	Larynx elevates below tongue base and tilts behind tongue.
Contraction of tongue base	Tongue is retracted backward, and bolus move away from the airway.
Epiglottis	Epiglottis is retracted by thyrolaryngeal tendon and turns over vestibule.
Vallecula	Bolus move in two way around the entrance of vestibule.
Swallowing apnea	Respiratory movements stops during swallowing.

Table 1.5 Organs with valve function for swallowing

Lips	make positive pressure in oral cavity
Soft palate	prevent flow to nasopharynx
Vocal cord	protect lower airway
Ventricular fold	protect lower airway
Upper esophageal sphincter (UES)	prevent reflux from esophagus
Lower esophageal sphincter (LES)	prevent reflux from stomach

b) Transfer of Bolus

The pharynx which was pressed and pulled in the transverse direction will spread in the front upper part, when the larynx carries out on elevation. Tongue moves by styloglossus and hyoglossal muscles, presses and pushes bolus, and proceeds it to the pharynx via isthmus of fauces. Although most of the bolus pass through piriform fossa, part of the bolus passes over epiglottis. Pharyngeal wall becomes shortened by lower constrictor muscle of pharynx, constrictor muscle above the bolus contracts, and bolus passed through entrance to esophagus. It is transported by the ring-like peristalsis.

In normal swallowing, the prompt transfer of bolus from mouth to stomach is possible. Liquid bolus passes pharynx within 2 seconds, and reaches to stomach in about 5 seconds. Transfer of the bolus is based on the motion by the muscle contraction and the gravity. Muscle contraction makes the portions of negative and positive pressure, and makes bolus transfer efficiently. This serial pressure formation is efficiently formed with lips, velum, vocal cords, and UES/LES at the time of swallowing (Figure 1.6, 1.7). A tongue forms the first positive pressure. Movement of tongue to lower back causes the elevation of larynx and hyoid bone. The elevation of larynx makes negative pressure in pharynx, and transports bolus from positive pressure to negative one safely. It is abnormal that bolus moves to a portion which is originally in positive pressure and results in penetration and aspiration.

D) Examination for Dysphagia: Evalvation System for Aspiration Risk

HAZOP analysis is performed to find out all the risks comprehensively (by Guidewords and Deviation) and to take measures (Layers of Protection) in each process of swallowing movement. In this section, an outline is summarized about the method of inspecting as a detection system for dysphagia.

1) VFSS and FEES (fiberoptic endoscopic evaluation of swallowing)

VFSS can evaluate bolus passage condition and can also observe motion of swallowing related organs. It cannot be overemphasized that VFSS is the gold standard for evaluating ingestion and swallow function, while it is also the fact that the VFSS result is not always in accordance with actual ingestion and swallowing condition. VFSS enables observation of not only the existence of aspiration but functional abnormalities of a swallowing related organs. Thus, the result of VFSS applies for deciding rehabilitation methods, route of feeding, texture of food, and posture during swallow. Since VFSS can observe swallowing movements of each phase, abnormalities can be found easily.

In FEES the abnormalities of larynx and pharynx, the existence of residue, and vocal cord function can be seen directly under accepting reality on real time, although the moment of swallowing cannot be seen (white out). The greatest advantage of FEES is its portability, and it can use at bedside. Since there is no radiation contamination as side effects, examination can be performed repeatedly. However, sufficient cautions are required for nasal bleeding and vasovagal reflex (syncope). FEES incorporated with sensory-function testing (FEESST: fiberoptic endoscopic evaluation of swallowing with sensory testing) is also reported.

The significant correlation between VFSS and FEES is reported for pharyngeal residue (80% to 92%), aspiration (84% to 100%), and penetration (85% to 86%). In addition to two kinds of this standard examination, combination of electromyography, tongue pressure measurement, and swallowing pressure measurement is also reported.

2) VFSS and other examinations for dysphagia

There are a few standardized questionnaire forms as dysphagia screening method, and they are reported in a self-entry type, a care worker entry type, and a medical staff entry type. The questionnaire (modified Fujishima Questionnaire) which we are using in our hospital revealed a specific pattern with different neurological diseases. The ideal questionnaire needs following three points. First, items consists of easy questions for patients, families, care workers, and medical staff, and result should not be influenced by experience of evaluators. Next, questionnaire could apply directly to daily meal and rehabilitation, if it contains an item about concrete ingestion and swallowing scene. It is also possible to offer the data which can respond to patient's swallowing training, foods creation, meal scene in a ward, and rehabilitation by a speech therapist. Furthermore, it becomes reference for the family and the care worker to make a meal at home. The third point is that the feature and severity of dysphagia can be judged to some extent.

Swallowing function is evaluated by voice change, dysarthria, cough after swallow, dysphonia, laryngeal elevation, and condition of saliva at a bedside.

Furthermore, although the correlation with aspiration is not shown, abnormality in pharyngeal reflex (gag reflex) and decrease of sensation in pharynx and larynx are reported to correlate with dysphagia. Though RSST (repetitive saliva swallow testing) is simple methods at bedside, there are few reports for applying RSST in deglutition disorders. It is reported that RSST decrease with the stability of a jaw. Although there are various reports about WST (water swallow testing), the volume of water varies according to reports. DePippo reported that 3-oz WST correlates with coughing during or after swallowing and wet voice in comparison with VFSS. Moreover, in Timed Test of drinking 150ml water, which measures the time and the number of swallow, revealed that dysphagia is correlated with extension of swallowing time, cough, and dysphonia. Daniels analyzed laryngeal elevation, the character of voice, and a cough at the time of swallowing water of various quantity. When two or more in six items (dysphonia, dysarthria, decrease of spontaneous cough, cough after swallowing, decrease of pharyngeal reflex, and voice change after swallowing) existed, abnormal findings were presupposed by VFSS.

About evaluation of aspiration, VFSS, FEES, swallowing pressure measurement, pulse oxymeter, and scintigraphy are reported to be practical. About the above-mentioned inspection, it is reported that swallowing in unnatural state may be seen under examination condition, and variation is in the reliability between persons (interobserver reliability) and the reliability in a person (intraobserver reliability). Moreover, there is also a report that significant difference does not come out in pulse oxymeter.

3) Evaluation of Central Control for Swallowing Movement

About the central-nerves mechanism of swallowing movement has yet to be uncovered, although the analysis is reported with fMRI, magnetoencephalography (MEG), or PET. Activated area associated with swallowing is reported in primary sensorimotor area, supplementary movement area (SMA), insula, operculum, parietal lobe, and temporal lobe. Furthermore, there is a report about the activity change under voluntary swallow (command swallow, volitional swallow) and reflex swallow (non-command swallow, natural swallow).

Functional brain imaging is classified into two methods; detecting an electrical activity of the neuron itself (MEG and EEG) or a change of cerebral blood flow accompanying neuronal activity (fMRI, PET, and fNIRS). The latter is based on the theory that the brain blood flow will increase in the region where the activity increases. Since change of the amount of blood is delayed to actual neuronal activity, the time resolution of fMRI is an order of a second. Because swallowing movement perform within 700ms, time resolution of MRI is relatively low. On the other hand, in MEG which can catch cerebral electric activity directly, analysis is possible at the time resolution of milli-second order.

Moreover, in our research the brain functional activities in swallowing movement can be measured by functional NIRS (near-infrared spectroscopy). The NIRS measurement by optical topography equipment is useful to the brain performance analysis of the ingestion and swallowing movement accompanied by operation which free posture can take. Our results indicate that brain activity is widely activated by volitional swallowing compared to reflective swallowing, and that movement of tongue, and of pharynx was separable with the difference of NIRS signal strength, and these results are in line with the previous reports by fMRI in a supine position. About the result of the NIRS signal pattern at the time of ingestion and swallowing movement, the application to the evaluation of function of swallowing difficulty and rehabilitation is expected.

E) Risk Analysis by HAZOP

As surveyed in this chapter, swallowing movement is controlled by the complicated process, and the risk management is not easy, either. Then, we considered HAZOP analysis to be the optimal method as the risk-analysis technique of swallowing difficulty. Table 1.6 represents the correspondence of the example of application in dysphagia with HAZOP sheet. Refer to the medical treatment HAZOP of Chapter 2 and Chapter 4 for details. The fine management of HAZOP analysis is attained with an inquiry of a risk more detailed as it enforces with a view from pathophysiological side to actual clinical care.

Table 1.6 Definition of HAZOP terminology in dysphagia analysis

Node, Subnode	each swallowing phase and more detailed process
Guideword	possibility to happen (or not to happen)
Deviation	abnormality in swallowing movement
Effect	results such as aspiration and pneumonia
Cause	Cause or mechanism of each deglutition disorder
Classification of the frequency	frequency of each deglutition disorder
Risk classification	significance of each disorder
Classification of the effect	contents of the effect of each disorder
Who	medical staff who is responsibile to check
Safety measure	examination for checking disorder

References
1) Crary M & Groher M. Introduction to Adult Swallowing Disorders. Butterworth Heinemann. St Louis. 2003.
2) Miller AJ. The Neuroscientific Principals of Swallowing and Dysphagia. Singular Publishing Group, Inc. San Diego. 1999.

Medical HAZOP

Chapter 2

A) HAZOP (Hazard and Operability Study)

Although various check list systems are created for risk assessment in dysphagia, it is difficult to inquire rare or hidden risks. Hazard and Operability Study (HAZOP) is one of the risk management tools for evaluating risk source. HAZOP is the method that the Chemistry Industrial Association (CIA) in Britain first published officially as CIA HAZOP Study Guide in 1974. It is an inquiry system of risks and track records, which accumulated for 30 years of history. Nowadays, HAZOP is applied to various industrial fields.

In this chapter the feature of HAZOP as a technique of an inquiry of a risk and applications of HAZOP will be introduced.

Many conventional accidents have occurred in the situation where a change (a change of design, a change of a procedure, a change of directions, etc.) is not correctly managed with. The risk inquiry technique should be selected to manage a possible change.

From the view of causes and results, the feature of HAZOP system is to determine several deviations and to analyze the results which occur from combined causes (Table 2.1). Thus, HAZOP is a system-based analysis tool which can clarify rare

Table 2.1 Methods for risk assessment and cause/ result

Mehod	Cause	Result
Checklist	casue=checklist	check=result
Fault Tree Analysis (FTA)	multiple causes	one result
Failure Mode and Effect Analysis (FMEA)	one mode	multiple results
Hazard & Operability Study (HAZOP)	deviation with multiple causes	multiple results

causes and rear effects systematically. Checking the accident which occurred in the past can be also included.

1) Overview of HAZOP analysis

HAZOP analysis aims at identifying the hazard of a process and the problem on operation.

The basic concept of HAZOP analysis is to investigate deviated process from normal status under a designed condition. If deviation from the original designed process condition arises, a possibility that the problem and the accident on the operation will come out. When an analysis team evaluates the cause and its influence by HAZOP, a guideword and a process parameter are used. These guidewords and process parameters are compared and contrasted with the process parameter which applies and corresponds to the specific point and specific section of process, and the possibility of the gap from predetermined condition is identified. The greatest strength of HAZOP analysis is being able to produce creative and innovative ideas by the brainstorming by members with various career. For this reason, it is important to create circumstances where members can exchange opinions freely.

2) Preparation for HAZOP

Although data required for preparation of HAZOP varies with scale and complexity of an object plant, data required for a general target is referred to the Piping & Instrument Diagram (P&IDs), a flow sheet, a plant arrangement plan, an operations manuals, a logic control figure, a logic diagram, or a computer program. A plant manual and an operator manual may be needed depending on the case. It is demanded for data to be exact and to be comprehensive. In the case of the existing plant, P&IDs should be checked, be updated, and is in agreement with the present condition, and the correction after plant construction is described in the drawing.

In the case of the chemical plant, most information is indicated by P&IDs. But in analysis of a human factor, it becomes possible to determine easily in HAZOP to set the node with role of a person according to the Work Breakdown Structure (WBS). Creating WBS is critical to perform analysis of all manufacture processes and operating processes by HAZOP (Table 2.2).

Table 2.2   An example of WBS

Node No.	Main Work	Person	Subwork	Problems and incident cases	Points to be paid attention
Inspection-1	Work1	Operator	Preparation for inspection (describe contents with timeline)	List up the point that mistake would happen in preparation and collect incident cases.	Describe the point to investigate
			Inspection work (describe contents with timeline)	List up the point that mistake would happen in inspection and collect incident cases.	Describe the point to investigate
		Inspector	Assessment of inspection	Judgment of a failure below the standard of decision	Standard of decision

3) Organizing HAZOP team

Usually, HAZOP study is performed in a multidisciplinary team, and members are selected based on the knowledge and specialty about design, operation, inspection, maintenance, and safety control. These days, a member well versed in the regulation applied from a viewpoint of legal compliance may be needed. Usually, it may be considered as 4-to 7-person organization, and every member has to have knowledge sufficient to the predetermined operation conditions of a plant.

It is important that the team leader is also skilled in HAZOP technique. Team leader has a role that members could observe to practice HAZOP. Therefore, a team leader is usually equipped with communication skills to command the staff who is not his subordinate, and thus the leader should be a talented person who can also pay careful attention to a subtle point. A secretary is nominated in the team to record the contents in a meeting, and the document would circulate to members by the following meeting.

Probably, the team leader will be desirable to be the person without the close relation to the plant investigator. Sometimes a technical contribution should not be expected from a leader, although sufficient technical knowledge which leads study appropriately is preferable for a team leader. It is effective for a team leader with prior training on the HAZOP technique.

4) Performing HAZOP study

HAZOP study is performed by concentrating on a specific point, a specific section, or a specific operation stage of process called "a node (a study node)." The range of a process targeted by one study may determine according to experience of a team leader. It evaluates individual line or vessel most ordinarily. If the team leader of HAZOP study is well experienced, two or more lines in one node could be included.

HAZOP team investigates each node and specifies condition deviation of the process which may lead to disaster. The intention of the design is checked in order to clarify the purpose and process parameter of apparatus first. It is determined by comparison and contrast of keywords a deviation and main process parameters whether the process has deviated from ordinary conditions. The key for a successful HAZOP study depend on effective use of keywords. Therefore, keywords should be defined clearly to put it into practice and its usage among all the team members.

a) Process keywords (Primary keywords)

The keyword mentioned here is related to operation situation of design intention of process or object plant. The main process-related terms are listed below, and the following list is an object for reference to the last. According to the target plant, keywords should be decided to use by evaluation (Table 2.3).

For example, probably some members think it unreasonable that "corrosion" becomes a keyword in a design phase, since corrosion of unexpected site should not be intended at the time of plant planning. Although almost all plants are designed bearing in mind a certain amount of lifespan, and unintentional corrosion must not be tacitly generated in a designed intention, it is assumed that occurrence probability must not exceed a fixed level. Therefore, when a corrosion rate of incidence goes up under a certain situation, it will be called a deviation from the design intention.

Table 2.3 Process Keywords (First Group)

Flow	Temperature	Pressure
Level	Isolation (settle, filter, centrifuge)	Composition
Reaction	Mix	Attenuation (grind, crush)
Absorbance	Corrosion	Erosion

Considering that a word "operability" is contained in HAZOP, the necessity of adding the operation-related term to the above-mentioned keyword will come out.

The keyword of the second group is overlooked and considered not to be so important (Table 2.4). As a results, for example, a plant operator will take a thoughtless procedure which may lead to disaster, since the safe interception method is not directed, in order to perform repair, peripheral equipment is temporarily made into off-line. Moreover, since the manual release procedure of the safeguard is not directed, it can be judged during a test run that a plant cannot be operated.

Table 2.4 Process Keywords (Second Group)

Isolation	Drainage	Ventilation
Purge	Inspection	Maintenance
Start-up	Shutdown	

b) HAZOP Guidewords (Secondary keywords)

We can point out a possibility of deviations and problems combining the primary and secondary keywords listed blow (Table 2.5).

In HAZOP study, overt and covert problems become clear by combining keywords and guidewords systemically. More concretely, combination of process keywords and HAZOP guidewords are performed.

Tabe 2.5 HAZOP Guidewords

Keyword	Meaning
No / None	Not achieved (example: flow/no), not done (example: isolation/none)
Less	Decrease (example: pressure/decrease)
More	Increase (example: temperature/increase)
Reverse	Opposite event happens (example: flow/reverse)
As well as	Achieved but other event happens (example: flow/association of pollution of the flow)
Other than	Unexpected event happens (example: flow/leak at unexpected area, composition/unexpected mixed ratio of materials)
Fluctuation	Achieved only temporally with fluctuation (example: flow/air rock in the pipeline)
Early	Early in timing or out of order
Late	Opposite to early

Although it seems that the scenario of disaster cannot usually be considered, explosion and the fire accident of the large-scale tank have occurred on the jet fuel accumulation base in Britain in December, 2005 (http://news.bbc.co.uk/2/hi/uk_news/4520430.stm). It is supposed that neither safeguards which should function essentially, nor measures worked. This accident taught us the following lesson: even if there are already the safeguard and the measure, we cannot ensure true safety without checking its functions correctly.

Analysis and evaluation procedure of HAZOP can be applied as flows, such as, a flow of thinking, and a flow of action, to an inquiry and evaluation of the risk of various fields by thinking as a process (Figure 2.1).

B) Medical HAZOP

The Japanese Medical Safety-Measures Review Committee submitted "medical safe promotion package of measures" in 2002 and stated as follows:

Reservation of medical safety has so far been performed in the responsibility of the individual medical doctor. For this reason, medical treatment is characteristic to be offered individually under a medical worker's technical knowledge and technology to the patient who has a different condition.

However, reservation of the medical safety of the system which was based on efforts of an individual medical staff, the system based on the medical technology and the knowledge for every conventional occupational description or specialty, is becoming difficult against the background of an advancement, complication of medical treatment in recent years, and it is necessary to improve the state of safety measures.

Medical service today is not supplied by individual doctor but by the system which consists of human resorce (multidisciplinary staff), things (medicine and medical instruments), organization (hospitals), and software. Even if anyone of these are unsuitable, service is not provided appropriately. For example, when medical treatment is offered by a team which consists of many occupational descriptions, if the rule in a team is inadequate or if there is not sufficient communication, it may develop into a medical accident. Therefore, it is a challenge

Chapter 2　Medical HAZOP　*31*

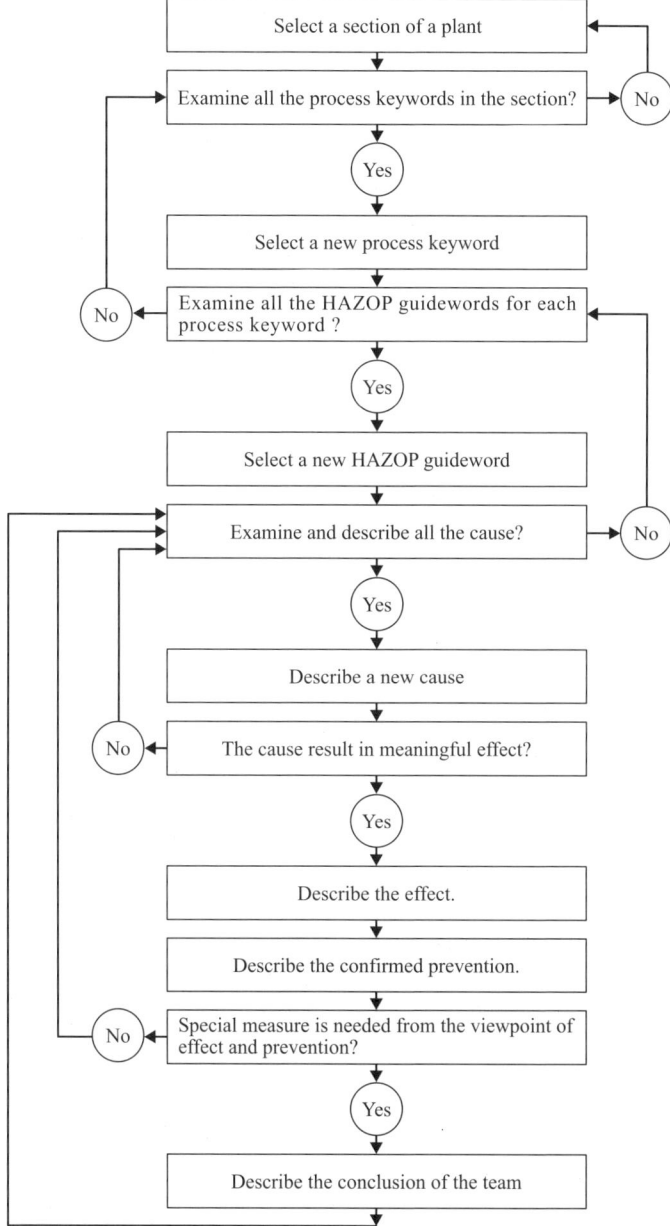

Figure 2.1　HAZOP Flow Chart

how the whole system perform safety in medicine, and how the quality of each element will be achieved.

In other industries, safety measures are already accepted with system-wide problem, and there are many examples under the advanced scientific technique. For instance, the improvement in the safety system by fail-safe (the system that does not result in disaster even if there is an error) or by fail-proof (error-proof, the system in which an error did not happen easily) is adopted in the manufacture industry in the technique of quality control of the product, in the nuclear industry, and in the airplane industry.

Although the system in other industries is not necessarily utilizable for medical area as it is, there are many points which should be considered as reference, such as having taken the systematic measure on condition of the thing which was a thin concept, and "for which people commit an error", and they need to take in such a technique at the medical spot from now on until now as positively as possible.

In addition, it is indispensable that all the related organizations are in agreement with each role assignment under cooperation, and tackle taking advantage of the position and capability while the medical institution which is the spot implements such a measure, respectively.

We tried application to analysis of dysphagia paying attention to the hazard operability study (HAZOP) technique in which it is used in the manufacture industry based on this measure from April, 2004.

1) Safety management system

The accident of each industry which occurred recently (outbreak of food poisoning in the food industry, death of the patient by malpractice in the medical industry, criticality accident in the nuclear industry, loan collection impossibilities in financial collapse, extensive disclosure of large-scale explosion and a fire, and a toxic substance in the chemical industry, trust loss in politics, and head-on collision in the railroad industry) are considered to be the worst result in each industry. These disasters are considered to be the result that the safety management system was not functioning.

It is our duty to construct the safety system so that such a maximum risk may not be occur.

The common causes of latest accident and incident are as follows;
− schedule priority
− sense-of-mission not wanting to inflict damage on an organization
− missing of raising a question which is not checked and reconsidered
− not to carry out according to the procedure and standard
− decrease of a sense of maximum risk
− miscommunication between an employee, a cooperation company staff, and an organization
− misjudgment of the administrator
− different situation as usual (state of urgency)
− not to reconsider the past accidents or incidents
− wrong success experience (nothing occurred by violation of a rule)
− decline of the procedure, the education, or the governance for risk management

Those who took this book in their hand would like to carry out the self check of whether such a thing has broken out first. The guideline and indicator about a safety management system of a certain form are created in all countries. However, in Japan examination of the measures based on the scenario in consideration of the enforcement procedure and worst case of risk assessment about a process have been rarely performed systematically.

That is,
− Risk assessment is carried out about an operation, a present construction project, and present materials/product, to specification of a potential risk for man, equipment, operating loss, community, and environment.
− Pinpoint the dangerous place and presume the damage (shown qualitatively first) and the accident frequency rate (shown qualitatively first) at the time of the occurrence of an accident. Next, the measure against prevention/mitigation for managing a risk continuously is drawn up and implemented.

- It is the point that periodical risk assessment should be carried out by the member including suitable specialists who is not related to the examince (a parent company and a specialized agency with evaluation capability).
- Risk assessment should be carryed out, when the defined interval has passed and when change arises.
- A evaluated risk is judged by the manager of each section, and determined matter must be documented clearly.
- Carry out an internal audit for structure and function of the system.

According to the important item demanded by the safety management system from such a background, the safety control system for medical facilities was created.

Process safety management is imposed by the regulation from the 1990s in US and EU as a safety control system to operate a petrochemical plant safely. The item and the contents of enforcement which are listed there are not peculiar to a petrochemical plant, and can be applied to all business conditions as a common safety control system.

That is, if we define a series of process with various practice for the medical purpose as a medical process, a medical-process safety management system is required as a management system for ensuring medical safety. The required item of the process safety management system both in process-oriented chemical industry and in a medical-process safety management system in the clinical settings are summarized in Table 2.6.

Although the medical-process safety management system consists of the following 15 items, many of them are performed in conventional education. (1) safety control plan, (2) organization and responsibility system, (3) safety control by medical staff, (4) medical safety information, (5) medical-process risk assessment, (6) medical practice and management of medical support system, (7) medical-facilities management, (8) education of medical personnel, (9) management concerning change of diagnoses, prescription, and treatment, (10) investigation of incident and major accident, (11) correspondence to the state-of-emergency, (12)

Table 2.6 Comparison of Process Safety Management in industry and medicine

	Indusry	Medicine
1	Leadership and safety guideline	Leadership and safety guideline
2	Organization and responsibility system	Organization and responsibility system
3	Safety management by workers	Safety management by medical providers
4	Information of process safety	Safety information (complication, contraindication)
5	Risk assessment (deviation from normal operation)	Risk assessment (deviation from normal treatment)
6	Management of operation and work	Management of medical procedure (clinical pathway)
7	Management of facilities	Management of facilities, information, and utility
8	Education of workers	Education of care providers
9	Change management (facilities, operations)	Change management (facilities, operations)
10	Investigation of accident	Analysis of incident reports
11	Emergency measures (mass destraction)	Emergency measures (incident/accident above 4b)
12	Risk communication (administrator, subordinate/ residents)	Risk communication (doctor, patient/care provider)
13	Management of the documents	Management of the medical chart, incident reports
14	Inspection	Inspection
15	Regular inspection of the system	Regular inspection of the system

risk communication, (13) documentation management, (14) audits, (15) periodical reexamination of systems.

Among these items, (5) medical-process risk assessment, and (9) management concerning change of diagnoses, prescription and treatment, (10) investigation of incident and major accident, (11) correspondence to the state-of-emergency, (12) risk communication, are thought to be important for preventing major medical accidents.

2) Medical-Process Safety Management System (MPSMS)

A medical accident can roughly be divided into two. One is a case caused by a doctor in their procedures. In this case a defense layer is the judgment of a doctor and the procedure itself. A different result may be followed by a moment act of a doctor. In order to prevent it, two or more defense layers are inherent in a doctor. A subtle mistake may cause a critical result in the medical practice performed in the situation where he/she is not conscious of two or more defense measures. It is because the doctor himself does not know that a small mistake may lead a big accident continuously.

Other case is caused by a malfunction of a systematic medical practice currently performed as clinical pathway in medical team. In this case, two or more defense layers exist and a medical worker and medical equipments can prevent a medical accident as protect layers.

The 5th item included in a medical-process safety management system; implementation of risk assessment is the contents which were lacking uniquely in conventional medical education. Although incident report contain the major accident more than 4b, risk assessment is evaluated according to a series of processes about incident below 4a. (Table 2.10)

However, if 15 items shown in Table 2.6 are not managed as a system, risk assessment could not be performed nor functioned correctly. 15 items of contents included in a medical-process safety management system are shown below.

Medical process safety management system (MSMS) contains 15 items of the following.
1. Leadership and safety control policy: The top of a medical organization must show medical safety control policy, and this should be performed and evaluated as a management system.
2. Organization and responsibility system: Each member should be aware of their role and responsibility for the management of a serious risk on total level of organization. Specific training for risk management should be specified, and regulation of training must be implemented. Participation of an employer and a subcontractor in a suitable case is also needed.
3. Safety control by medical worker's participation
4. Safety information : The contents about medical facilities, complications, and contraindications of medicine must be summarized as manuals or standard documents. It is important that the item of "9. Change management" should be corrected exactly.
5. Risk assessment: This portion is equivalent to risk source specified in the notification No. 86 from Japanese Administration of Economy, Trade and Industry and OSHA/PSM. In order to analyze the cause and measure on deviation from

regular medical practice or a state, solution would be conducted by a checklist system, What-if system, FMEA, HAZOP, ETA, FTA, or risk matrix evaluation. While the checklist is effective in analysis of procedures where the change is not made, HAZOP is effective in analysis in the act and the state where changes occur. Risk assessment specifies systematically a serious risk of producing from normal or unusual situation, and it carries out the adoption of procedure which evaluates the degree of seriousness, the possibility of the accident, and the influence of the risk.

6. Medical facilities, medical information system, and utility management: Grasp medical facilities, information system, and the advance level of degradation and damage by periodical inspection, evaluate a result, and check having the reliability to which these equipment and a system can be equal to continuous use. Repair/replacement maintenance based on inspection method and interval degradation/damage evaluation is also included.

7. Adoption and enforcement of procedure about safe medical institution management should be performed including maintenance at time of skill maintenance of medical worker, medical information system, medical equipment, and temporary business suspension.

8. Education of medical personnel

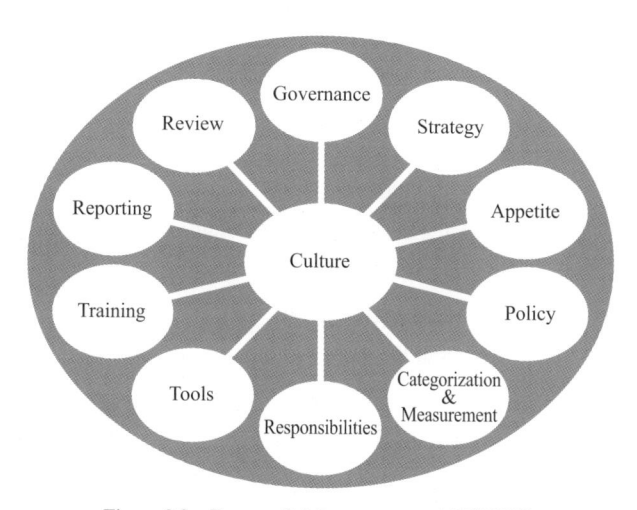

Figure 2.2 Frame of risk management (BS31100)

9. Change management (diagnosis, prescription, and medical treatment):

When partial change of diagnosis, prescription, and medical treatment, or complete change have done, implementation of common knowledge thoroughness procedure of contents of change should be performed. In business, it is the most important part. It is ctirical to be managed in the form in which record contains with the form of 5W1H. Objects are changes of all the items shown here and reflection of an evaluation result, and they are candidate for HAZOP analysis. The major cause of the big accident or the everyday accident of all fields reveals to be insufficient change management.

The objects of change management are standards and equipments (medical equipment, ward equipment, medical information system), which required for management of medical facilities, and a medical worker. It must be evaluated and managed so that it may fit in the level which the risk of safe and health produced by these change as small as possible. Therefore, the following systems should be formed and functioned. When a change is made, it is also important that risk assessment is carried out according to risk assessment procedures, such as HAZOP.

The system which manages both temporary and lasting change should be formed and is functioning.

The system for management of change needs following factors:
− Authorization of admission of change
− Analysis on safety, health, and environment
− Observance of the rule and the recognized standard
− Acquisition of the permission needed
− Document including the reason for change
− Common knowledge about the degree of a potential influence and the measure needed for the results
− limitation of duration
− training

It ensures that a temporary change does not exceed the recognized original range or an original period without examination or recognition.

10. Investigation and analysis of incident reports: When an accident occurs, investigation conducted in order to clarify the cause of an accident and to prevent a recurrence. Although the cause of an accident is often reported as human error, if the primary cause (root cause) for the human err is not clarified, another accident will occur repeatedly. Only by the FTA technique, the primary cause could be clarified. Implementation of analysis and evaluation which combined What-if, ETA, HAZOP is also needed.

11. Plan of management for emergency: Possible risk will be clarified with systematic analysis, and the procedure which conduct preparation, examination, and inspection for specifying to the crisis should be chosen and performed in order to prevent from the risk. In the state of emergency in the clinical settings or an organization, is it possible to clarify in advance the role of the measures and person in charge, who makes the scale of the damage reduce. It is important to perform a simulation and an exercise in everyday life and to raise the capability corresponding to the state-of-emergency.

12. Risk communication: Medical risk is located under the circumstances where staff says the following comments, "It must have been pointed out before", "from which having meant is not transmitted", "as for wrong interpretation", and "wrong belief".

There is a risk in the communication between a doctor and a patient, a doctor and a medical worker, and a medical worker and a cooperation company employee's.

13. Documentation management: To carry out risk management, it is also important that the monitoring of the enforcement situation is carried out by internal audit, that the system and the organization will make an improvement according to the advise for the problem, and that there are documents which have accountability.

Moreover, all the items should be recorded on a documentation management system, and the latest version after change must be managed, and these procedures should be announced to the medical worker.

14. Monitoring of performance: If all the process leaves unfinished, a management system does not function. The contents of enforcement and the improvement of business are evaluated according to all the items of 1 to 13 listed above, and an improving point will be pointed out and performed if there is a problem. These evaluation cycles should be repeated and carried out. Adoption and enforcement of procedure which evaluate continuously the conformity to the target which the medical institution management person's major accident prevention plan and medical safety control system (MSMS) are needed. Mechanism of investigation, and the mechanism of the correction measure when not working is also needed. Suppose that the system of the medical-facilities management person who reports the near mistake of a major accident, especially the malfunction of measures, and the ex post facto measure based on near mistake investigation and its teachings are included in procedure. (It is a subject for a hospital manager and a general risk manager)

15. Audit and inspection: This is adoption and enforcement of a periodical systematic evaluation procedure about the validity and conformity of a medical safety control system (MSMS). Creation and updating of an inspection document about this plan by a senior executive, and the performance function of a medical safety control system shown. The correspondence which linked these to the documentation management system or the information system is needed. (Subject for a hospital manager and a general risk manager)

3) Medical-process risk assessment

As foregoing paragraph showed outline of 15 items included in a medical-process safety management system, the methodology of medical-process risk assessment is described here.

Medical practice is an aggregate of various medical processes, and is realized by the teamwork of the medical worker of each field. For detailed application example will describe in Chapter 3.

According to UA OSHA 29CFR.1910.119, the Compliance Guidelines and Recommendations for Process Safety Management (Non-mandatory), the purpose of this section is to introduce the created medical-process risk assessment:

(1) Medical-process risk assessment (MPRA) is called medical process risk assessment, and it is the most important item of a medical-process safety management system.

(2) MPRA is the technique of enumerating probable serious risk, and analyzing risk factors, and evaluating these risks and risk factors systematically in medication which may cause the act and the critical sequela of a doctor or a medical worker.

(3) The result of risk analysis and evaluation which became clear by enforcement of MPRA should be shared by the medical workers, make safety system more active at the time of execution of medical practice and medication, and make a medical worker perform a judgment which can reduce an unexpected bad influence.

(4) MPRA analyzes and evaluates the result and the cause of medical practice, an accident, and enforcement of procedure.

(5) Analyze and evaluate MPRA at a narrow sense about the flow of steady business and the flow of unsteady business about doctor and medical staff, patient, medical equipment, medical information system. Although it was required for the wide sense to examine the external factor which may have influence above, the interpretation in a narrow sense was adopted here. MPRA is a method which clarifies a risk of lurking in a medical process.

4) Process analysis for medical procedure

In analysis of various risks of lurking in medical practice, it is required to clarify the element which divides medical practice into every process and role. In the industrial world, the method called Work Breakdown Structure (WBS) on the occasion of a plan and execution of a project has been widely used as fundamental method for project management. This method can be utilized when creating a clinical pathway. Commercial project management software can also be used.

By making WBS, the roles of a doctor, a nurse, a pharmacist, an engineer, medical equipment, and medical information system utility are clarified, and the information of the stage and the duration that they participate and of the skill which they required would be shared. The example of WBS sheet is shown in Table 2.7.

In the industrial field, the WBS information is prepared as drawing and

Table 2.7 Work Breakdown Structure (WBS) Sheet

Harvard Manage Mentor - PROJECT MANAGEMENT TOOLS
Work Breakdown Structure

Develop a Work Breakdown Structure (WBS) to ensure that you do not overlook a significant part of a complex activity or underestimate the time and money needed to complete the work. Use multiple pages as needed.			
Describe the overall project:			
Major Task	Level 1 Sub Tasks	Level 2 Sub Tasks	Level 3 Sub Task Duration
Total Duration (minutes/hours/days/weeks)			

(From Harvard Manage Mentor on Project Management)

specifications (Piping & Instrument Diagrams: P&IDs) in the design phase of a process.

Although medical workers, such as a doctor, a nurse, a pharmacist, and an engineer, originally know what should be done with each role (motion and function of a stationary state). Here, an understanding as a team can be advanced by clarifying what should be done with a role, and by identifying a role of the defense layer (preventive measures).

5) Inquiry of incident report for analysis and an accident example

While creating above-mentioned WBS, technique and empirical rules of procedure are described by the point of a problem and a work. Furthermore, the description of the subnode, where an incident and an accident occur, advances HAZOP enforcement smoothly. It is desirable for these information to be able to pull out from a medical information system.

6) Medical HAZOP

As for enforcement of the medical HAZOP, it is desirable to divide into two types to carry out. First targets are the incidences above 4a, whose frequency is rare but whose effect is large (Table 2.10). One example is the operation which a doctor conducts. Another is a inpatient care whose frequency is high but whose effect is comparatively small. Dysphagia corresponds to the former and the latter.

As Figure 2.3 shows the Heinrich's law, serious accidents can be analyzed by HAZOP analysis, and it becomes possible to analyze even the middle-scale accidents and incidents. On the contrary, a possibility that analysis of a serious accident cannot be reached from the number of cases in the analysis from incident reports is high. As shown in Figure 2.4, HAZOP analysis considers the result from a deviation from the stationary state and speculates various causes (human, environment, equipment, and exterior) indirectly and conducts the analysis for incidents below 3b.

The influence, which occurs when gap arises from the regular medical act compulsorily according to a basic guideword, is considered also in medical HAZOP. A secondary guideword is shown in Table 2.8; this is the same as secondary general guideword. The difference of HAZOP used in the medical field is only primary guideword for medical terminology.

The guideword "No/None" means not to carry out (or unable to do) the purpose or the act. If it does so, you have to consider the cause which is not carried out (or it cannot do).

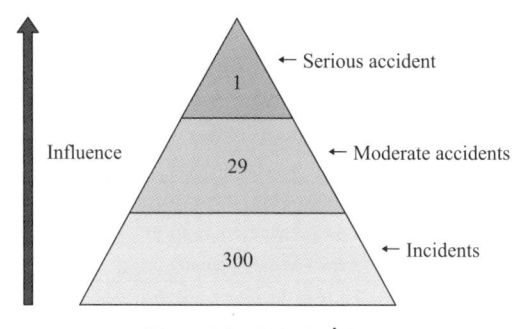

Figure 2.3 Heinrich's law

44

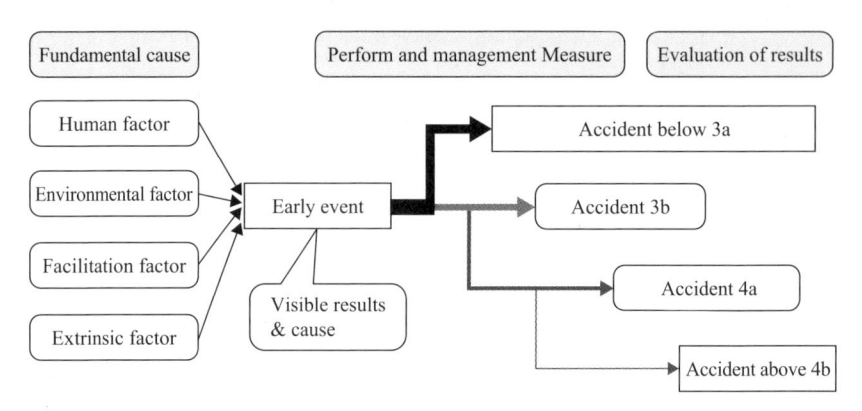

Figure 2.4 Objectives and procedure for HAZOP

With the guideword "Less", we can consider that an act is inadequate and is not attained with the purpose. Similarly, we have to consider the cause for it.

Creation of WBS and a series of accompanying procedures select and combine primary guideword, and support creation of a deviation scenario. The deviation scenario of HAZOP is created combining the product of subwork (primary keyword) and the secondary keyword shown in Table 2.8, which described the contents of the medical process. For example of central venous puncture, since an act and a procedure peculiar to this technique are explained from the WBS sheet, deviations in the act in the basic node of local anesthesia are listed, which kicks the puncture act (primary keyword) in the stationary state shown here by combining with the

Table 2.8 Basic Guidewords (secondary keywords)

Deviation	Meaning
None/No	Not happen: denial of intension
More	Quantitative increase above limit or standard
Less	Quantitative decrease below limit of standard
Reverse	Opposite event happens
As Well As (AWA)	Achieved but other event happens
Other Than (OT)	Unexpected event happens
Part Of (PO)	Achieved only partially
Early	Early in the timing and misjudgment
Late	Late in the timing and misjudgment

Chapter 2 Medical HAZOP 45

basic guidewords. A basic node can be divided, the check of an local anesthesia ⇒ diagnostic puncture ⇒ puncture ⇒ check of the catheter position.

The important point for performing medical HAZOP is to consider deviation according to basic guidewords, based on the performance procedure normally performed according to the main nodes in the medical treatment and medical system. Deviations can be easily considered from incident reports or experience of medical experts. Eaven though incidents which the participating member has not experienced or accidents which nobody knows could not imagined, deviations can be created mechanically according to basic guidewords. As long as the created scenario is theoretically possible, the deviations should not be deleted from the candidates for examination. Thus, it becomes possible to clarify the rare cause of an accident. The example of the medical HAZOP sheet which added improvement is shown in Table 2.9.

Table 2.9 HAZOP Sheet

Code No	Guidewords	Deviations	Effect 1 Event 1	Frequency	Cause	Person	Measure
A-BC-001	Select from None		Event result from deviation	often (1 per Month)	cause of deviation	doctor	examination for deviation
A-BC-002	Less	Make deviation scenario	Event result from deviation	sometimes (1 per year)	cause of deviation	doctor	examination for deviation
A-BC-003	More OT	from subnode in WBS	Event result from deviation	often (1 per Month)	cause of deviation	nurse	examination for deviation
A-BC-004	AWA R		Event result from deviation	seldom (1 per several years)	cause of deviation	doctor	examination for deviation

7) Evaluation with risk matrix

From the results of medical HAZOP in medical procedure or incidents we can evaluate the significance of the risk with risk matrix.

To prevent medical accidents it is important to decrease an incident below 3b (Table 2.10), however, it is also needed to decrease one above 3b from the viewpoint of social influence. According to the result in HAZOP, when the effect of 4b happens, the risk position is located in C, D, or E according to the frequency. Classification of

Table 2.10 Level of medical accident/incident in Japan

Risk Rank	Degree	Duration	Report	Contents
5	deadly injured		accident report	death caused by accicents
4b	seriously injured	continuous	accident report	serious injury which remains continuously
4a	moderately injured	continuous	accident report	moderate injury which remains continuously
3b	seriously injured	temporarily	accident report	serious injury which needs procedures and recovers
3a	moderately injured	temporarily	incident report	moderate injury which needs procedures and recovers
2	lighty injured	temporarily	incident report	injury which does not need procedures
1	no	no	incident report	incident happens but cause no harm to a patient
0	no	no	incident report	incident do not happens to a patient

Table 2.11 Classification of frequency

Classification	Definition
Highly Frequent	several times in a month
Frequent	several times in a year
Occational	once in several years
Uncommon	once in ten years
Remote	once in twenty years
Rarely	once in a future

frequency is shown in Table 2.11.

Figure 2.5. represent a matrix with two axis: consequence and frequency of a risk. Category A to E refers to the priority to take measure. Although if it seems that the accident of the same incident level 4b, measures must be immediately taken for one occurred "frequently", while for one occurred "seldom" or "low" to perform reexamination of a safeguard or a measure periodically are possible measures. It becomes possible to assign limited resources (a man, a thing, and gold) to the large measure against an accident of an effect by performing such evaluation. As a result, while becoming possible to reduce the accident more than level 4b, it is a level 4a by the analysis peculiar to the medical treatment HAZOP like an event tree. It can carry out by combining the measure against the following incident report levels.

Chapter 2 Medical HAZOP 47

Risk Rank

Level	Remote	Uncommon	Occational	Sometimes	Frequent	Highly frequent H	Highly frequent HH	Highly frequent UH
Level 5 Deadly injured	D	D	E	E	E	E	E	E
Level 4b Seriously injured	C	C	D	D	E	E	E	E
Level 4a Monderately injured	B	B	C	C	D	D	E	E
Level 3b Seriously but temporally injured	A	A	B	C	C	D	D	D
Level 3a Moderately and temporally injured	A	A	A	B	B	C	C	C
Level 2 Injury without procedures	A	A	A	B	B	B	B	C
Level 1 No harm to patients	A	A	A	A	A	B	B	B

	Remote	Uncommon	Occational	Sometimes	Frequent	Highly frequent H	Highly frequent HH	Highly frequent UH
	Once in 20 years	Once in 10 years	Once in several years	Once in a year	several times in a year	once in a month	once in a week	once in a day

Frequency

E	Need a prompt measure to take
D	Proceed safeguard and procedure
C	Regular inspection of safeguard and procedure
B	Reannaunce of safeguard and procedure
A	Keep ongoing safeguard and procedure

Figure 2.5 Risk Matrix

HAZOP for Swallowing Disorders

Chapter 3

1) Preparation for HAZOP

As shown in Chapter 1, the swallowing process is classified according to the function, and evaluation has been performed according to the swallowing phase. The main nodes and the subnodes according to the function for the swallowing process are shown in Table 3.1. HAZOP was carried out for every subnode listed below.

The HAZOP for dysphagia shown below is created according to the motion of bolus that is the foundations of swallowing process. In this chapter, the node of pharyngeal phase will be shown. In addition, examples of application are shown in chapter 4, which include surgical procedures, human factors, rehabilitation methods,

Table 3.1 Nodes and subnodes in swallowing process

Node No.	Main node	subnodes
SW1	Recognition Phase	Understand food and start ingestion
SW2	Preparatory phase	Ingestion and mastication to form bolus
SW3	Oral phase	Tongue moves bolus to oral canal
		Bolus contacts Wassilief area to start swallowing reflex
		Bolus end passes through oral canal
SW4	Pharyngeal phase	SW4.1 : Soft palate attaches tightly to pharyngeal wall
		SW4.2 : Tongue and palate shut tightly to prevent from oral reflux
		SW4.3 : Larynx elevates
		SW4.4 : Epiglottis falls
		SW4.5 : Vocal cord closes
		SW4.6 : UES opens
SW5	Esophageal phase	SW5.1 : UES closes tightly
		SW5.2 : Bolus moves with peristalsis
		SW5.3 : LES opens

clinical pathway, in-home care, and medical research.

By illustrating to a matrix, understanding for the risk is obtained shown below.
(1) There are risks with both harmful effect and high frequency in the matrix. These risks need to be corresponded immediately.
(2) The effect of the risk becoming more harmful as deviation increases. There are two types of growth of the risk; the risk that increases gradually with deviation step by step, and the one which jumps to a high level of danger with a little deviation.
(3) The incident whose effect increases gradually, can be observed and taken measures with a time to think over.
(4) The risk increased abruptly with a little change of deviation, should be corresponded immediately, and checking system for the risk must be clarified.

When there is much amount of bolus, or when texture is unsuitable, inflow to the larynx and aspiration can occur. The following can be considered as a measure for dysphagia. The quantity which a patient puts into a mouth needs to be managed (with the explanation and the education to a patient and a family about proper quantity of bolus) for the case with suitable texture management in an inpatient's meal. The quantity which a patient puts into a mouth needs to be managed for the case who takes a between-meal snack.

2) Pharyngeal Phase

Pharyngeal phase can be divided into five more subnodes.

SW4-1: Bolus comes to tongue base and larynx begins to elevate. At the same time velum contacts posterior pharynx wall and closes nasopharynx to prevent bolus from reverse to nasal cavity.

SW4-2: When bolus passes, tongue base, the velum, tongue, and hard palate stick completely, and adverse current into mouth will be prevented.

SW4-3: Respiratory tract entrance is narrowed with laryngeal elevation.

SW4-4: Epiglottis falls.

SW4-5: Epiglottis closes.

HAZOP was carried out for every subnode listed above. Hereafter, the influence, cause, and frequency accompanying typical deviation are analyzed for every subnode.

3) Subnode 3 (SW4.3) in Pharyngeal Phase

Analysis with deviation guidewords are listed in Table 3.2 in Subnode 4.3 (SW4.3). Among them a deviation of LESS are described as "Since elevation of pharynx is inadequate, tracheal gill is not closed. There are clinical examples which exists in mostly elderly people." Table 3.3 indicate results when Less deviation occur. The

Table 3.2 Deviation in SW4-3 (Laryngeal elevation)

Code No.	Secondary guidewords	Contents of deviation
SW4.3-01	None/No	Larynx does not elevate, and airway does not completely shut
SW4.3-11	Less	Larynx does not elevate completely, and airway does not completely shut
SW4.3-28	Delay	Larynx elevates with delay, and airway does not completely shut
SW4.3-41	Slow	Larynx elevates slowly, and airway does not completely shut
SW4.3-51	Delay & Slow	Larynx elevates with delay and slowly, and airway does not completely shut
SW4.3-61	Less & Slow	Larynx elevates incompletely and slowly, and airway does not completely shut
SW4.3-71	Less & Slow	Larynx elevates incompletely and with delay, and airway does not completely shut

Table 3.3 Deviation of Less in SW4-3 (Laryngeal elevation) : analysis of effects and cause

Code No.	Deviation	Effect 1	Effect 2	Effect 3	Effect 4	Cause
SW4.3-11	Larynx elevate incompletely (Less)	Bolus goes to lower pharynx				Disease of cerebrum Disease of medulla or cranial nerves (IX, X, XI, XII) Disease of muscle Disuse Aging Oral or pharyngeal cancer
SW4.3-12		Bolus goes to laryngeal entrance (penetration)	Remove bolus			
SW4.3-13						
SW4.3-14			Aspiration	Remove all		
SW4.3-15				Remove partially		
SW4.3-16						
SW4.3-17				Remove partially	Pneumonia	

Chapter 3 HAZOP for Swallowing Disorders 51

influences, cause, influence level, and measure to take are entered in the HAZOP sheet. An evaluation result is also shown in these tables.

In the next step, each codes are evaluated by frequency and impact of the risk. As shown in Table 3.4, this deviation has many clinical examples, dysphagia occurs every day, and there is a case which results in pneumonia. It is important to recognize that dysphagia occurred frequently (everyday), and the risk of pneumonia increases when a part of aspirated material is not discharged.

Table 3.4 Deviation of Less in SW4-3 (Laryngeal elevation) : analysis of frequency and impact

Code No.	contents	Results	Frequency	Impact
SW4.3-11	Bolus goes to lower pharinx	No harm	Frequent UH (several times in a day)	B
SW4.3-12	Bolus goes to larynx	Check by exam.	Frequent UH (several times in a day)	C
SW4.3-13	Bolus removed	Check by exam.	Frequent UH (several times in a day)	C
SW4.3-14	Aspiration	Treatment	Frequent HH (once in a day)	C
SW4.3-15	Remove all the bolus	Treatment	Frequent (several times in a year)	B
SW4.3-16	Remove part of the bolus	Treatment	Frequent HH (once in a day)	C
SW4.3-17	Remove part of the bolus ⇒ aspiration pneumonia	Treatment Intensive care	Frequent H (once in a month)	D/E

4) Information from HAZOP Analysis

Risk rank distribution is shown in Table 3.5 for every evaluation scenario of the node of oral phase, pharyngeal phase, and esophageal phase in HAZOP. Although the evaluation result of all the scenarios is distributed over A or B ranks in oral and esophageal phase, distribution of C or more ranks appears in pharyngeal phase. In a deviation with elevation of larynx and closure of respiratory tract entrance, distribution of D and E ranks is also accepted. Although it was known that pharyngeal phase is critical for the swallowing function, HAZOP analysis revealed that the risk in the subnode of elevation of larynx and of closing of respiratory tract is high (Table 3.5).

HAZOP-SW-5.4-1
Risk Rank

Elevation of epiglottis and closure of air way

Risk Level	Remote	Uncommon	Occational	Sometimes	Frequent	Highly frequent H	Highly frequent HH	Highly frequent UH
Level 5 Deadly injured	D	D	E	E	E	E	E	E
Level 4b Seriously injured	C	C	D	D	E (pneumonia)	E	E	E
Level 4a Monderately injured	B	B (pneumonia)	C	C (pneumonia)	D	D	E	E
Level 3b Seriously but temporally injured	A	A	B	C	C (not clear)	D (clear a part)	D	D (not clear)
Level 3a Moderately and temporally injured	A (clear all)	A (clear a part)	B	B	C (aspiration)	C	C (not clear)	
Level 2 Injury without procedures	A	A	A	B (clear)	B (aspiration)	B	B	(claer) Larynx does not elevate enough, and air way does not close ⇒penetration (12) ⇒flow to pharynx (11)
Level 1 No harm to patients	A	A	Larynx does not elevate, and air way does not close. ⇒ penetration (2) ⇒ flow to pharynx (1)		B	B	B	

Ellipse numbers: 26, 20, 24, 17, 7, 9, 25, 6, 8, 23, 16, 19, 22, 15, 4, 14, 5, 3, 13, 2, 10, 1, 11, 12

Frequency scale:
- Remote: Once in 20 years
- Uncommon: Once in 10 years
- Occational: Once in several years
- Sometimes: Once in a year
- Frequent: several times in a year
- Highly frequent H: once in a month
- Highly frequent HH: once in a week
- Highly frequent UH: once in a day

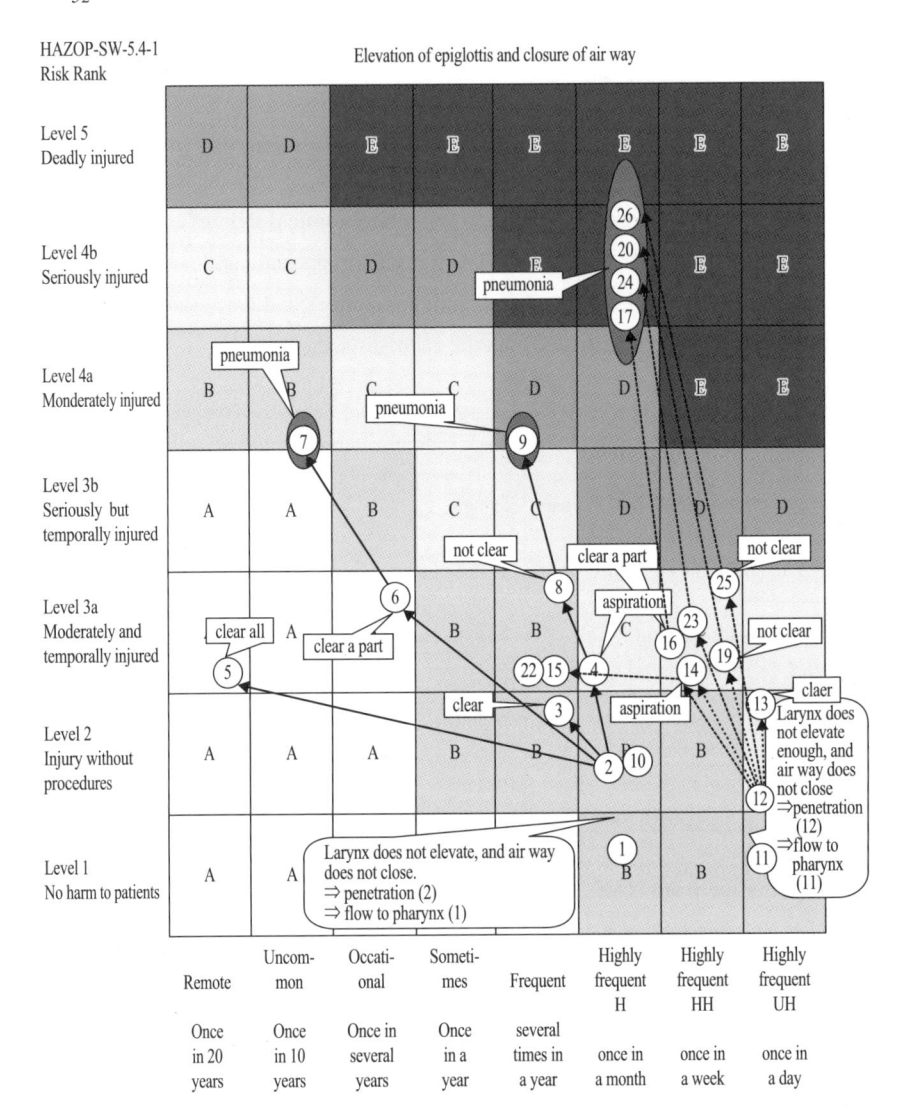

Figure 3.1 Risk Matrix in SW4.3-1

Table 3.5 Analysis of risk rank in each node

Node No.	Main node	Contents of nodes and subnodes	Risk rank A&B	C	D	E
SW3	Oral phase	Tongue moves bolus to oral canal Bolus contacts Wassilief area to start swallowing reflex Bolus end passes through oral canal	100%	0	0	0
SW4	Pharyngeal phase	SW4.1: Soft palate attaches tightly to pharyngeal wall	65%	35%	0	0
		SW4.2: Tongue and palate shut tightly to prevent from oral reflux	92%	8%	0	0
		SW4.3: Larynx elevates	55%	31%	7%	7%
		SW4.4: Epiglottis falls	79%	21%	0	0
		SW4.5: Vocal cord closes	100%	0	0	0
		SW4.6: UES opens	100%	0	0	0
SW5	Esophageal phase	SW5.1: UES closes tightly	100%	0	0	0
		SW5.2: Bolus moves with peristalsis	100%	0	0	0
		SW5.3: LES opens	100%	0	0	0

Application of HAZOP for Risk Management in Dysphagia

Chapter 4

4.1 Medical HAZOP in Clinical Settings

A) Challenges for medical accidents

From 1999 the distrust to medical treatment came to spread among people in Japan caused by the occurrence of big medical accidents, such as patient picking mistake at operation at Y University and death accident by injection of the antiseptic to venous route in the Metropolitan H Hospital. Medical safety and safe reservation has been important subjects for medical community with progress of the medical science and medical technology. Various medical safety measures are implemented in all the hospitals regardless of size, and medical safety organization came to be evaluated also in the medical insurance. Collection of incident cases started in October 2001, the "Medical Safety Promotion Package of Measures" was published in 2002, and all the medical institutions are asked to offer safety medical treatment by the Ministry of Health, Labor and Welfare.

However, on the other hand, the report about a medical accident still continues, and sometimes criminal liability is imposed on the persons involved in an accident as a recent trend. Although the medical institution side has not necessarily neglected the measure for safety, the fact is that an accident is reported scandalously. Therefore, the distrust to health care grew severe further, and the situation is also born, which medical staff cannot concentrate on the cooperation with a patient collaborate and fight to diseases.

Then, what is the problem of the safety measures of a medical institution in Japan? As already stated, there are 29 slight accidents in the shadow of one serious accident, and it is supposed that there are 300 incidents in the base further. If a serious accident occurs in fixed probability from incident, to prevent a major accident it is necessary for us to reduce an incident first.

Based on this view, also with the incident without actual harm, it reported as incident reports and various improvements have been practiced in the medical institution. In the industrial field, it is equivalent to what is called TQM (total quality management) and QT (quality control) activities. Example of the result of this are colored syringe for external-application and pre-filled syringe of potassium chloride (KCL). Moreover, a double-check system is performed in many scenes, and wearing of a wristband which prevents patient misconception is performed in the hospital. As a result of such efforts there is an opinion that the simple mistake, called human error, will never cause a major accident from now on.

The subjects which still remain are "the care on medical treatment" and "the medical treatment and procedure" performed by doctors. Although the care on medical treatment is an unclear classification, fall accident in a hospital and suffocation by dysphagia at the time of meal are included in this criteria. There may be a limitation in preventing unexpected fall or aspiration by the number of the present limited nurses, and it may be difficult to reduce these incidents only with TQM or QT activities. In this book, a new view is shown for the purpose of the preventive measures of dysphagia.

1) Lessons from the report

According to the "outline of the accident" in 2006, there are 152 accidents result in death and 201 in serious side effect in one year (Table 4.1). Though total of 353 accidents are the same amount as ordinary year, it is important for improvement of medical safety to reduce the number of death and side effects. Of course, it seems that many inevitable complications are included in this number in addition to the accidents based on a doctor's negligence. However, efforts to decrease such kind of complications will be demanding from now.

According to the classification of contents of accidents, 152 cases (46 death and 96 side effects) are categorized in "medical treatment and processing", and this is the most frequent cause which medical doctors associate. Others are 94 affairs (61 death,

Table 4.1 Contents and degree of accidents in 2006 (Japan)

	Death	serious aftereffect	mild aftereffect	unknown	not selected	total
Ordering	0	0	10	3	0	13
Medication	2	8	47	20	0	77
Bood transfusion	1	1	3	2	0	7
Medical procedure	46	96	234	70	4	450
Medical apparatus	10	11	65	29	0	115
Examination	6	5	47	14	0	72
Care	26	46	230	37	0	339
Other	61	33	95	33	0	222
Not selected	0	1	0	0	0	1
Total	152	201	731	208	4	1,296

33 obstacle survival), and fall and swallowing accident follow the next.

Furthermore, according to the investigation of the situation where accidents occur (Table 4.2), the most frequent situation were open-abdomen or open-thorax operations, followed by endoscopic treatment and vessel catheter medical treatment. There are only two accidents of central venous puncture and only two of transfusion relation affairs. Although there are not a few accidents by the intravenous injection or oral medicine agent, the category of "medical treatment and procedure" has exceeded others. Based on this result, regardless of mistake serious affairs depend on medical treatment/procedure associated with medical doctors rather than incorrect medication or transfusion. It seems that comparatively simple mistakes, such as variant transfusion, anesthetics, and overdose of potassium, decreased considerably by conventional safety activity. Taking these situations into granted, in order to improve medical quality, it is a big challenge how to reduce the risk in medical treatment regardless of mistakes.

2) Lessons from national survey

Japanese Anesthesia Society reported a national survey on accidents during anesthetization. According to this report, among 536,000 times of the examples of anesthesia investigated in 1998, 7.32 cardiac arrest happened by accident and 4.04 death per 10,000 cases. The cardiac arrest rate of incidence due to anesthesia was

Table 4.2 Site and degree of accident in 2006

	Death	Serious aftereffect	Mild aftereffect	Unknown	Not selected	Total
Medication and Injection						93
preparation of medicine	0	1	5	0	0	6
injection (subcutaneus, muscle)	0	0	4	2	0	6
intravenous injection	0	3	11	5	0	19
arterial injection	0	0	1	0	0	1
intravenous drip infusion	1	1	12	5	0	19
central venous catheterization	1	1	2	3	0	7
oral medication	1	2	10	3	0	16
nasal, eye drop	0	0	2	0	0	2
drug delivery with other methods	1	3	3	0	0	7
preparation of oral medicine	0	0	3	3	0	6
preparation of injection medicine	0	0	0	1	0	1
other	1	0	1	1	0	3
Blood transfusion						7
blood type	0	0	1	0	0	1
method of transfusion	1	1	2	2	0	6
other	0	0	0	0	0	0
Medical procedure						402
open-head	2	3	6	2	0	13
open-lung	1	8	6	4	0	19
open-thoracic	2	2	6	2	0	12
open-abdomen	6	6	28	2	0	42
limb	1	3	4	0	0	8
endoscpic operation	1	5	16	2	1	25
other operation	1	13	27	12	0	53
preparation at preoperation	0	1	0	0	0	1
procedure at preoperation	1	1	2	0	0	4
postoperation	4	3	8	2	0	17
other related with operation	2	6	16	5	0	29
general anesthesia	0	0	2	2	0	4
local anaethesia	0	1	1	0	0	2
inhaltation anesthesia	0	0	0	1	0	1

intravenous anesthesia	0	1	0	0	0	1
spinal anesthesia	0	0	1	1	0	2
other associated with anesthesia	0	0	0	0	0	0
Caesarian operation	1	1	4	0	0	6
other operation of obstetrics	2	3	4	0	0	9
dialysis	2	0	7	1	0	10
IVR (catheter therapy)	1	4	15	5	0	25
radiation therapy	0	0	3	2	0	5
rehabilitation	0	0	2	0	0	2
dental procedure	0	0	1	0	0	1
endoscopic procedure	5	3	15	3	0	26
other related with therapy	0	8	17	8	0	33
central venous line	2	0	12	4	0	18
peripheral venous line	1	0	3	0	1	5
dialysis line	0	0	0	1	0	1
feeding tube (NG・ED)	0	2	0	0	0	2
urether catheter	0	0	0	0	0	0
drainage	0	2	3	1	0	6
treatment of injury	1	2	0	0	0	3
other associaed tubes	1	0	9	2	0	12
intubation	0	1	1	0	0	2
tracheotomy	1	0	0	0	0	1
cardiac massage	0	0	0	0	0	0
oxgen therapy	0	0	1	0	0	1
other associated with emergency	1	0	0	0	0	1
Medical apparatus						43
mechanical ventilator	2	2	2	1	0	7
oxygen generator	0	1	2	1	0	4
artificaial cardiopulmonary	0	0	0	0	0	0
cardioversion	0	0	0	0	0	0
pacemacker	1	0	0	0	0	1
infusion pump	0	1	1	1	0	3
dialysis pump	0	0	2	0	0	2
EKG, BP monitor	0	0	0	0	0	0
pulse oximator	0	0	0	0	0	0
other appratus	2	3	19	2	0	26

calculated 0.88 per 10,000 examples, and mortality rate was about 0.04. 31.0% of the cause of cardiac arrest is made from the human factor, the accident which medical staff associate. The incidence of cardiac arrest during anesthesia is only 0.01% or less, and the ratio of it is one to 10,000, however, we must consider the fact that the incidence of cardiac arrest caused by human factor which can be prevented with an effort, happened one to 250,000 times.

It turns out that the measure about the medical accident which unripe environment, such as an error of apparatus and medicine, already developed mostly, and it became a time aiming at how the accident resulting from doctor's own technology or diagnosis could be reduced. In the case of experienced doctor, there are more problems of the lapse of judgment in intentional selection or technology itself than incident. That is, in order to reduce medical accidents further, I think that the necessity of cutting directly is in the medical quality, apart from the work which reduces incident based on Heinrich's law.

Absolute liability may be asked even if it is innocent. There is a view that it causes withering medical treatment and never induces useful directivity to a patient, and, the view, in which it is humbly reconsidered by one side whether all the complications are really inescapable, will also be important.

3) Quality of medicine,

The medical worker always aims at high quality medical treatment based on conscience. Then, what is the constituent factor of "the medical quality"? Probably it is just the high quality medical treatment itself to offer advanced medical treatment specially, and it is also an element in connection with the "quality" as service business not to cause the simple mistake in injection and medication. Moreover, the height of the amenity of the whole hospital and the number of acceptance of emergency care also serve as elements which determines the quality of a medical institution.

Three outcomes (result), "safety", "good quality", and "satisfaction", are needed for the medical quality. If a good result is obtained safely, it can imagine easily that a patient's degree of satisfaction increases. If it is the same disease, in addition to it, duration of hospitalization can also be managed for a short period of time, and

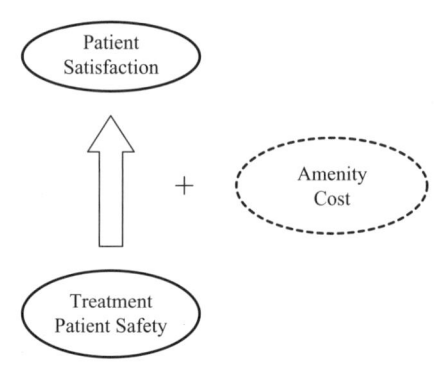

Figure 4.1 Factors influencing medical qualiy

the medical treatment which can be passed safely and comfortably will turn into the highest quality medical treatment during hospitalization. It would be carried out more cheaply, in addition, if possible (Fig. 4.1).

Recently the treatment results of medical institutions have come to be compared in our country. For example, treatment results can be exactly compared about specific cancer by five-year survival ratio. Furthermore, it is higher quality to be fewer complications, if probability of survival is the same. It is reasonable that not only with complications but medical accidents could be avoided. However, even if a medical institution with quite sufficient quality on the average, a final result does not necessarily become uniform for individual specificity. It is the nature of what is called "medical uncertainty." About this "medical uncertainty", it supposes that "The medical treatment can essentially become uncertain and possibly harmful for patients, because life is the nature of finitude, complexity, and diversity." in a doctor's conduct code defined in Toranomon Hospital. That is, even if the medical staff offers uniform medical treatment, a result is not uniform since the reaction to it varies with individual patient.

From the patient side, all the medical treatments he receives may come out one and only, and it may be thought that the word "medical uncertainty" is only an excuse by the side of health care providers. To one aspect this comment sounds reasonable. Comment from the side of medical care providers "Results may differ even if we offers the uniform medical treatment of the highest level." It becomes a standard of judgment how it is for itself as a side to receive. Then, the medical provider side must also make the preparations which can respond to the needs by the side of various patients. However, a patient's reaction to simple medical practice is also too variable in fact, and it is impossible to correspond to individual cases.

Also about a medical accident, the excuse of "having brought a different result since the patient's reactions differed, although it was generally presupposed that sufficient medical treatment was performed" is often used in such a background. "Although we underwent an operation by predicting it as a local area, however, since it was large lesion in fact, bleeding increased more amount than anticipated, and transfusion was not in time." is a good example. In such a case the patient side has the question whether the preparations for the worst case were anticipated, or why the worst case scenario was not predicted. The excuse by the side of medical providers for this may become "It is impossible to prepare for the complications which rarely happen, because it takes time, effort, and economical futility." If it sees from the side of medical economics, it may not be unreasonable, but as for patient side, asking for the highest preparation is reasonable. Then, it is necessary to take between both and to prepare for the worst case as considerable as possible. Even if special medicine or transfusion are not actually preparing for the worst case, a simulation for the correspondences to a possible accident only by bearing in mind will help themselves. It is a fundamental view to maintain quality against uncertainty of medicine.

4) medical accidents and medical malpractice

It is a wish of all the medical staff to reduce the number of serious medical accidents as low as possible even if medicine is uncertain in nature. According to Table 4.2, most serious medical accidents have occurred in operation or examination. It is a seriously illness patient originally who needs an operation or an invasive examination and results in unsuccessful. However, on the other hand, in many such cases, the boundary between an avoidable medical accident and an inevitable complication becomes ambiguous. Although a doctor's negligence is not allowed to be intentionally concealed under the name of complications, the avoided accident may also be included in what is made into complications.

The accident in such an operation or an examination procedure are not resolved only by the improvement of the system by TQM (nature management of synthetic) based on incident reports. This is because a patient's safety in medical treatment or examination is dependent not only on the safety of a system but the judgment and skill of doctors who are as the last executors. However, a doctor does not consider only safety in the first place, and does not necessarily choose the final decision for diagnosis or procedure. When there are several choices in patient's medical treatment, contention of a risk (danger) and a benefit (profits) occurs and, finally the probability of success and failure actually serves as a basis of determination. The difference to take a risk arises by the method of the recognition to the safety of the doctor or the medical team. Furthermore, a philosophy and a skill of an individual doctor are also considered. In addition to the factor by the side of health care providers, factors of the patient side, such as a patient's individual specificity and a view over a patient's own medical treatment, are also influencing. The end products differ in the following situations: to choose the operation with great risk aiming at complete remission, or to choose one with low risk bearing incomplete remission. In the accident produced under such a background, it can sometimes become ambiguous about the boundary of complications and negligence.

5) Medical safety management

One of the indicators for checking medical worker's safety consciousness is the number of incident reports. Incident reports are created when medical accidents or incidents occur, and they are used for finding out the defect on medical risk management system. it is regarded as a problem that reports from medical doctors are less than ten percent. Naturally the doctors who are busy working in the hospital, should also encounter incidents in a certain frequency. Among them there must be incidents related to serious medical accidents. However, probably because there is consensus of medical uncertainty among the doctor, there is also an atmosphere that a certain amount of accident is permitted. This is not a desirable situation, even if they are not indulging themselves.

From another viewpoint, Heinrich's report may not be believed by a doctor. It is necessary to reduce the adverse experience in the scene of medical treatment and procedure where a doctor involves directly, for realization of safe medical treatment, making full use of all methods. If the doctor does not believe Heinrich's report, we have to prepare the appropriate plan for a doctor. It is because an accident may decrease depending on how to keep the consciousness of the doctor as the last executor.

B) A model for developing safety management

Double-check and repeated practice are too simple for a doctor. It is necessary to prepare the policy which inflames intellectual curiosity to some degree. In a young doctor's education we should consider a systematic method rather than a simple one. Moreover, they need to be learned with advance consideration about how it is carried out in practice. It is clear that medical treatment is not performed by a doctor to a patient, or a nurse to a patient.

1) Medical science and health care

In order to consider the safety in the clinical settings, it is important to recognize a difference of medicine and health care first. Although health care means medical practice, the medical department is not enough for the education about "the state of clinical medical care." Medical education has been constructed to figure out the difference between normal and abnormal or health and disease according to organs basis. Recently there came criticism that the viewpoint of existence of patient as a human is missing, and importance came to be attached to the view of patient-centered medicine. The idea of patient-centered medicine is that a patient is treated as a human being, and that medical treatment must be considered as mental or social issues as well as physical. However, we think it inadequate that education how to carry out medical procedure to succeed a treatment and to keep patients healthy.

It is important to aware that many medical workers are participating to perform medical treatment for one patient in the hospital. The doctor needs to turn consciousness to existence of many medical workers. On the contrary, the medical practice which can cause an accident may also be brought by two or more medical workers. A doctor controls an act of the medical worker who has participated in simultaneously, and bears the role which the whole medical treatment advances smoothly while he is an executor of medical treatment. Each participant including a patient manages his role exactly, and it is essential for ideal medical treatment that information is transmitted correctly.

Of course, a doctor has decisive power and responsibility in serious medical practice or final judgment. In the previous medical accident, the doctor in charge and other doctors in prostate operation were attached only to new technical acquisition, and it was presupposed that they were lapsed into tunnel vision, and they lost control of loss of blood, and the timing of blood transfusion. Since the idea attained to only the impending role without the other participant being also conscious of the flow of the whole medical treatment, it might bring about the tragic result.

The responsibility for medicine is in the entire team which offers medical treatment. The chief executive in it is a doctor and fulfilling the duty links patient safely directly. For that purpose, being conscious of a team are required to grasp a medical flow.

2) Health care is a project for aiming at patient cure

"Project" is the activity performed in a fixed period aiming at achievement of a certain purpose. The target size and the period are not related to set the "project." In hospital the medical treatment to each patient figures out to be one project. In this meaning, all the medical workers should already be concerned with a certain project. For example, an operation is one project, and a subsequent chemotherapy is also one project. Some projects are put together to complete the medical treatment for one patient. One project consists of some processes. Therefore, in order to ensure the safety of each process the medical safety to a patient are needed.

In the industrial field, in order to make a project safely and successful in the manufacturing industry or in a service industry, process control is performed exactly. What kind of work is a project manager in the industrial world doing? They are management for progress of a project, negotiation with a customer or a user, management of personnel expenses or expense, reservation of the necessary personnel, and arrangement a report to the persons concerned. There are miscellaneous works, and they will be endless. Just by everything going smoothly, it leads to a success of the project which is a policy objective.

As the project manager in another field, doctor's role in medical treatment is in advancing a medical treatment process toward a policy objective called a success of medical treatment as well.

3) Medical HAZOP

In this book, management of swallowing is analyzed by the technique of HAZOP (Hazard and Operability Study), and the measures against troubles are shown. Among the risk management technique currently performed in the industrial world, Root Cause Analysis (RCA) and Failure Mode and Effect Analysis (FMEA) have so far been introduced in the medical community. The former is an ex-post analysis, the latter is an ex-ante-analysis tool, and it is used widely in the industrial field as the improvement-in-quality technique. Although HAZOP is also a tool for an ex-ante analysis, the feature is in the point of analyzing a dangerous factor according to guidewords. The excellent point of HAZOP is that the dangerous factor which exists in medical practice potentially can be comprehensively treated by guidewords.

RCA consists of creation of an occurrence flow chart, extraction of the problem according to analysis and creation of an unfortunate figure, and verification of a causal chain for the purpose of exploring the fundamental cause of a medical accident. Finally, the board of a hospital decides upon the measure to the primary cause.

FMEA is a method that performs brainstorming about a potential failure style and analyzes the influence after illustrates the process of medical practice. Unlike HAZOP, FMEA is not set guidewords for imagining a failure scenario in brainstorming, and offering all opinions anyhow is told as a key to a success in FMEA. Since there is no hint for deviation, a possibility that an opinion in brainstorming will be restricted to members' experience only, and it is less comprehensive in FMEA than in HAZOP.

Even if books on medicine has the statement of complications or side effects, it is rare to mention fully to the scene, act, and cause of occurring complications. Moreover, neither the human error which may involve as one of the causes, nor the error of equipment is indicated. They are under a principle that we must be infallible.

Although the serious medical accident by communication error between medical staff and a doctor may occur, it is outside a scope in this textbook. In fact as for most portion, the communication error is involving among incorrect medication. Actually the communication error between nurses resulted in incorrect venous injection of disinfectant in 1999. Such a direct cause is not written in the textbook, and only some complications in relation to a intervention may written in a textbook (Fig. 4.2, 4.3).

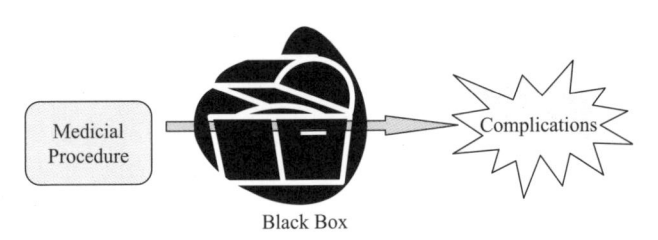

Figure 4.2 Black box of risks

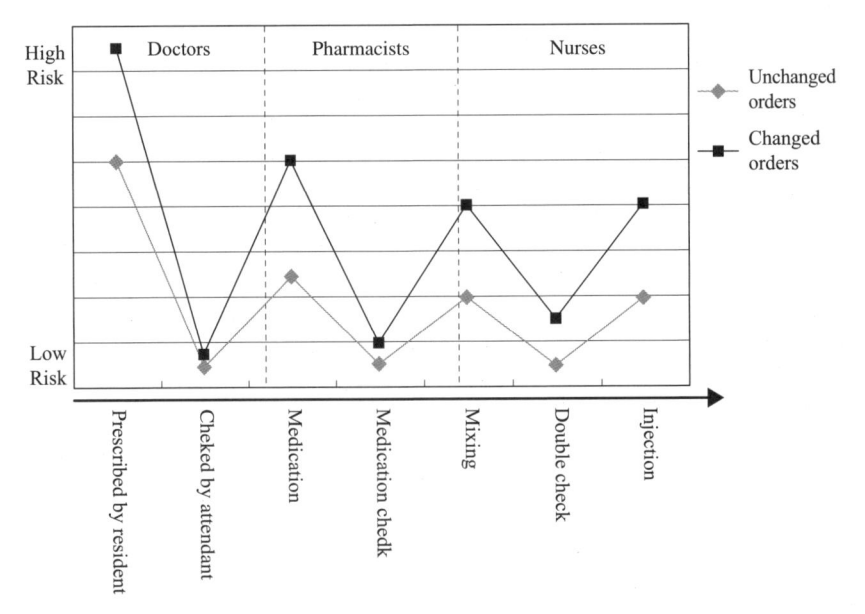

Figure 4.3 Risks from prescription to injection

It is the first step of accident prevention to grasp in advance what kind of trap is awaiting to each medical practice. Before complications or an adverse experience occur, the ways of coping to prevent should be prepared so that it may not have influence of to a medical treatment, that is medical project. It is risk management to elaborate a measure so that the influence may be minimized, even when it generates. For that purpose, We analyze a process of operation in advance, and think that the quality control technique which elaborates a measure supposing the dangerous factor which lurks there is effective.

C) Application of medical HAZOP
1) Safety education and medical HAZOP
With medical HAZOP, the process of medical practice is decomposed, a dangerous factor is explored by brainstorming, and it checks about the concrete measure further. This work of a series takes a remarkable long time. Although HAZOP are carried out several hours daily over a couple of week in the industrial field, there is not so much time in a medical community .An important point will be that a participant learns a HAZOP view and employs it efficiently in daily practice.

2) Management of medical process
Everyday medical treatment makes it a policy objective to regain the patient's health, and is advanced in the combination of various medical process. For example, medical process begins with medical interview and perform physical examination and laboratory investigation, and various medical staff will be associated with this process. After diagnosis is completed, medical treatment is started, but there are various choices, such as medication, injection, operation, and radiotherapy, With medical treatment, in order to regain health, each process is combined for every patient and it practices by choosing the best way for the patient. In this way, when we think about medical process, it turns out that each processes differ from every patient, and the process management which looked being the same as that of the industrial field is also difficult in medicine. Even if the final goal of every patient is health acquisition, process of every patient to reach the goal must be different.

Thus, it is impossible to cover all the risk to analyze with detailed HAZOP like a chemical plant. Therefore, in medical HAZOP, it is necessary to consider the medical practice which appears in one scene as one unit (module). Like the example of an operation shown abo☐e,decomposing and arranging a process may also contribute to safety, without carrying out to detailed ☐A☐☐☐analysis.

3) Analysis of condition

Like aspiration currently treated in this book, it is difficult to analyze a condition which one final result is caused by many factors. Although it is a cause that there are too many factors, it is also considered to be one of the reasons that the methodology for analysis is not established. ☐uch many factors can apply the ☐i☒v of the medical treatment ☐A☐☐☐also to the arrangement and analysis of a phenomenon which in☐ol☐☒ intricately.

(Example) Analysis for factors cause falls

☐a☒icipants: ☐urse leader ☐

E☐e☒t: falls

Time: 2 hour x 10 times

☐ackground: The accident in the care on medical treatment of an inpatient re☐☐eds to be the second frequent cause of death and serious sequela. Among them most frequent accident is falls.

☐a☒ses of fall accidents are basically patient factors, such as consciousness le☐el,physical inability, and dementia. ☐owe☐er, the medical institution could ha☐e the responsibility for offering safe hospitalization en☐ironment after e☐aluating a dangerous factor, as long as it was in the hospital. ☐h en femur neck fracture and intracranial hemorrhage occur due to falls, danger may attain to a life. ☐ easures should be taken for pre☐ening such kind of accident , since the purpose of a hospitalization aiming at medical treatment will be completely lost if it occur.

☐efore starting ☐A☐☐☐analysis, it is preferable to perform brainstorming on predictable risks, and a next session will become smooth in many cases. Although the opinions actually mentioned in the brainstorming about falls in Table ☐.☐it turns out that cause factors are summarized to se☐eral categories based on this.

Table 4.3 Risks for falls (brainstorming)

Site	Cause	Description
7th floor at night (vending machine area)	entangled, giving way	need to recognize as soon as possible using monitor camera
room at night	delirium	difficult to be aware by oneself
room at night	entangled, giving way	need to recognize as soon as possible by nurse call and sensor mattress
in the morning	entangled, giving way	frequent in the first action
in the morning elevator hall)	entangled, giving way	frequent in the first action
in the morning (toilet)	entangled, giving way	frequent in the first action
bathroom	slip	mattress for food
bathroom	uncontrole balance	when carer do not see
toilet	loss of consciousness	
toilet	uncontrole balance	when carer do not see
toilet	move beyond the power	when carer do not see
X ray room (outpatient)	entangled, giving way	unaware of a need for asistance
X ray room (inpatient)	entangled, giving way	unaware of a need for asistance
with visitor	entangled, giving way	when visitor do not see
with visitor	uncontrole balance	incorrect assisstance
with visitor	move beyond the power	unaware of patient ablitiy by oneself or carer
in psychiatric ward	hypotension	
in psychiatric ward	action together	accidents occur simultaniouly
in neurology ward	low ability of movement	effect of dementia
in neurology ward	delirium	difficult to be aware by oneself
in cardiac surgery ward	low ability of movement	effect of dementia
in cardiac surgery ward	entangled, giving way	need to recognize as soon as possible by nurse call and sensor mattress
in cardiac surgery ward	move beyond the power	unaware of patient ability by oneself

In the HAZOP analysis conducted on it, it becomes possible to assume various causes according to guidewords. Here, the horizontal axis was set as guidewords, and deviation was summarized for the scene and the environmental factor on the vertical axis for the time being.

Summary

1) In HAZOP analysis for endoscopic operation of hernia extraction, it was the purpose to mention the gap produced by the medical process in order and to get to know all the dangerous factors finally. Moreover, also by management of the medical process, medical practice was analyzed by the time series and it aimed the same at elaborating a measure in search of gap. Such usage is the same purpose as FMEA at the point of improving quality by finding a dangerous factor in advance. However, it seems that HAZOP using guidewords is excellent in the point that a dangerous factor can be examined comprehensively. Next step we showed that HAZOP is a useful tool for analyzing cases with complicated factors.

2) The greatest feature of the medical HAZOP is the point that it can search advancing analysis according to guidewords for a risk factor comprehensively. By using this feature, not only a mere ex-ante analysis but analysis of complicated pathology is enabled. In the domain of medicine or medical treatment, the view of HAZOP which treats the deviation from a process scenario is a very important and useful tool.

4.2 Risk Communication and HAZOP

A) Risk communication using risk matrix
1) Evaluation of human factor by HAZOP

After the accident of JOC which happened in Japan in 1999, the consciousness to the human error and human factor in the country increases. Human err has come to be related with the risk management and with the safe culture of a company or an organization.

Then, from the analysis of accidents and incidents in Central Research Institute of Electric Power Industry or the Tokyo Electric Power Co. Inc., the consciousness that the viewpoint "human error is not a cause but a result" is risen for taking the measure against an error. Since then there have been a body of discussion about the problem of the human factor in an accident broadly, and it has come to be understood also as a problem of risk management and safe culture.

It becomes to be important to eliminate direct/indirect factors (insufficient conditions in work environment, unsuitable man machine interfaces, a system that is not easy to use for man, the organization lacking safe culture) which cause human error, instead of blaming a person who has the responsibility for the accident. Professor Reason (Manchester university) who is a researcher (and also a psychologist) of the ergonomics of Britain, has presented the Swiss cheese model as shown in Figure 4.4 , noting that conditions for a systematic accident will be happen in the state where the hole of the wall of protection overlaps continuously.

That is, generally the accident do not happen according to one factor, but rather it will happen when many phenomena containing human error are connected in the state in an undesirable fashion. Several factors exist in the human error, which are successfully passing through each wall of a cheese slice of protection. Since one of the wall of the protection layer is a check by man, a human error arises when it goes wrong. Therefore, if it can stop with somewhere in walls of the defense, the view that a final accident is avoidable. This view is fundamentally the same idea of defense layer analysis (Layers of Protection). In this meaning, human error is one phenomenon which constitutes an accident, and it becomes important recognition that it is the "result" of being induced from a back factor from a viewpoint of error prevention.

The consciousness is risen that the viewpoint "human error is not a cause but

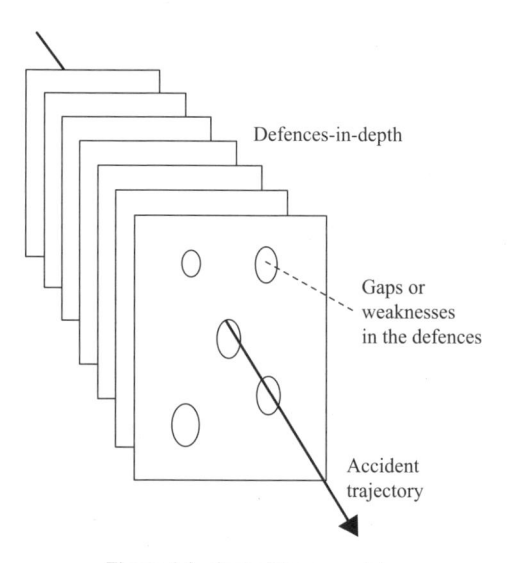

Figure 4.4 Swiss Cheese model

a result" works on the measure against an error ignited by a JCO accident, and discussion was made about the problem of the human factor in an accident broadly, and it has come to be understood also as a problem of risk management and as a safe culture of a company. The idea of a human factor is used from an aviation industry around 1970, and the basic model of a human factor has been proposed, corresponding to the purpose of risk management historically.

There are four models of human factor listed below. For details, please refer to another reference.

・SHEL model
・m-SHEL model
・P-mSHELL model
・4M4E model

The Ministry of Health, Labor and Welfare in Japan analyzes examples of accidents including the attribute of the personnel or a patient, the kind of accidents and incidents, and finds out information required for medical safety. Moreover, they checked the fact of an example and analyzed cases using various kinds of techniques to prevent generation and recurrence of medical accidents. Methods widely used in the medical institution about analysis of the accident are reported as follows.

http://www.mhlw.go.jp/shingi/2007/03/s0309-12.html

【Tools analyzing causes of accident 】
  (1) Root Cause Analysis (RCA)
  (2) SHEL model
  (3) 4M-4E
【Tools analyzing process and preventing accidents 】
  (1) Failure Mode & Effects Analysis (FMEA)

B) Category of human factor and HAZOP

About the classification of human factor researchers have discussed in the framework mentioned above, and they reach a consensus for defining human factor. In this section, Professor Komatsubara (Kanazawa Institute of Technology) is arranging the view of a classification of human factor with the measure against human error based on the latest example. According to his theory a person can be considered as the information processing system, and it is expected that the measure against human error is also demanded by understanding the limit and feature in the process of this system.

The arrangement and the measure against human error based on this view has been tackling in the field of ergonomics. From a viewpoint of the measure against human error, he defined three type of the error, an error of an individual, an error of a team, and a breach of the rules. This outline is shown below.

1) Error of an individual

There are limitation of the ability, feature of the ability, escape one's memory, shortness of knowledge and skill, and covert factor.

a) Limitation of the ability

Man's capability is expressed by the word of "power", such as "eyesight", "hearing ability", "judgment", "memory", "physical strength", "tenacity", and "capability of operation". By training, although it is possible to improve this "power", there is limitation in it.

The "power" of ordinary human being declines with a peak of 20 years old (aging). It is not avoided although there is individual difference. Therefore, if the work system was designed considering the youth as a premise, elderly people will be in a "misdirection-of-strength" state. Since the elderly people can respond to a capability fall by rich work knowledge and experience, the increase in human error is not immediately meant by aging. However, in order to avoid human error and to improve working efficiency, improvement of work system is desired so that work may be possible by less "power".

b) Feature of the ability

Error and lapse of memory is produced with the performance of capability. It is the feature that it cannot be answered why such a thing was done even if it blame the person who had human error. The classic example of this kind of human error is an optic illusion (geometric illusions). Even if the person makes cautions with an effort, it is hard to be improved by education and training. An error is generated also in a cognitive stage. Typical examples are mistake made in taking and misapprehension.

When two or more similar things are juxtaposed, or when there is time urgency, it is easy to produce a mistake. The reason of this is considered that humans tend to save time by skipping the check of a discernment issue, if the remaining time becomes small in order to avoid becoming work under-subscription. Moreover, since the consciousness to a discernment issue becomes thin, this kind of human error also tends to happen to the experienced person who works with a skill base. This is so called elementary mistake of a veteran, and incidents of medicine picking and a patient mistake in a hospital are equivalent to this.

A veteran may misunderstand, when he affected by his experienced in the past. It especially tends to be dragged by the case with much generating frequency. Although work generally progresses smoothly by using the past experience, when this backfires, this will also be called the elementary mistake which a veteran causes.

c) Lapse of memory

Lapse of memory means that the candidate for cautions shifts to another work and does not carry out the remaining portion of previous work in the middle of a series. Typically, one forget to carry out a subsequent work step when the main part of work is completed. Examples of lapse of memory are to leave a medical instrument inside the body and sutured a surgical operation or to forget to remove a instrument in repaired plant.

d) Shortage of knowledge and skill

Human error will happen easily If one do not have enough knowledge and skill required for work. It is true that a person who "cannot be carried out" or "does not know" is a problem, and the administrator is also a problem, who is taking out the person with insufficient capability and skill to the working place. Fundamentally, this problem will be solved by proper arrangement of the man-power or the necessary personnel with education and training.

e) Hidden factor

Even if the same person, the same work, or the same working condition may bring about human error. This is because the difference in a hidden factor for the reason.

There are the following hidden factors.

- what stimulates one's capacity for work may be reduced (a hand does not move by cold)
- what stimulates leaving wishes from work (hot, cold, stink, noisy)
- what reduces an awakening level (consciousness level) (fatigue, a medicine, predawn work)
- things which reduce motivation and morale (the work in which the purpose does not clarify, bad human relations, a low salary)

Such a hidden factor concerns workplace environment directly, and can be regarded as the object for risk management as an organization and as a problem of safe culture.

2) Error in team

There is a human error in an entire team by the problem of misunderstanding among team members from the beginning. If there are loss of communication or discommunication in team working or as succeeding work, it will lead to a fatal accident. It is unexpectedly difficult to take exact communication so that the accident in Yokohama City University Hospital occurred in 1999, and fault reliance and fault reserve may lead an accident whose responsibility locates in a team rather than an individual.

3) Breach of the rules

When the human factor is considered in the general industrial field, a breach of the rules occurs as one of the problems of human error. Although violation is different from the demanded performance to "deviation" and is human error in definition, it is intentional deviation and does not adapt itself to the word "human error." Violation can roughly be classified into "saving of work resource" and "self-satisfaction."

a) Saving of work resource

It seems that human being has a tendency to save the resources related to working time, effort, and expense. For example, it is thought that the following violations originated in this category.

(a) Omission: what is generated since a time-consuming procedure is skipped.

(b) Superfluous saving : altering the expiration date of food on purpose.

(c) The safety system as a foul trick

Although a safety system is equipment with the goodwill against emergency human error, it may be taken as the foul trick since it will not require time and effort compared with regular work sequence. Example for this category are the incorrect use of sensing device implemented with earthquake fire-extinguishing equipment of by having kicked away to a burner; the Shigaraki Kogen Railway accident (1991) which expected incorrect use of sensing device, and the train was left by the red signal.

Like a criticality accident of JOC, these misconduct is accelerated, when the company is in the climate of resource reduction (cost cut).

b) Self satisfaction

It generates, when an in appropriate procedure leads to satisfactory consciousness. The following is contained in this criteria.

(a) to do an excessive thing (one has the consciousness of being praised by the others)

(b) to make oneself look smart (the act of a "a slight hand" (a hand is taken out just for a moment, without suspending a machine at the time of a trouble) in the manufacturing industry: it has the sense of superiority that a measure can be taken without stopping a machine)

Various deviations are considered in the literature about these human error/human factor by reference. A patient, a doctor, a nurse, a speech therapist, and a dentist are concerning ingestion and swallowing disorders in the clinical settings. In this book we try to analyze the result and the influence of deviations from the regular work (a medical examination, instruction, rehabilitation) from a viewpoint of human error/human factor.

C) Human factors and guidewords in HAZOP

The example which related to a human factor extracted by brainstorming is shown below. These problems and causes have described from the cases which the participants concerned with and occurred every day.

As a problem in the side of health care provider
- laboratory findings is not understood nor informed in the team
- misdirection of procedure for care
- drug is not effective or wrong medication
- wrong belief/ones'own way
- inexperienced
- information is not shared
- lack of leader
- violation of a guideline or a rule
- oversight
- simple mistake
- timing is shifted
- bad atmosphere in the workplace

Applying the technique of HAZOP, combination with a secondary keyword will be considered as follows. As a result, it turns out that there are a problem previously taken out as shown in Table 4.4, a problem which must be taken into consideration besides a problem and a cause. The hidden problem can be clarified by creating HAZOP guideword from the listed problem.

As a problem in the side of a patient
- The gap between the goal of the rehabilitation and the hope of a patient or family
- inadequate understanding of pathology, examination data, and rehabilitation
- wrong method of taking care of a patient

Table 4.4 HAZOP guidewords related to human factors

Primary keywords	Secondary keywords	HAZOP guidewords
Understanding	· No/None	· do not understand the result
	· Part of	· understand part of the result
	· As Well As	· misunderstand the result
	· Reverse	· misunderstand as an opposite result
Medication	· No/None	· do not medicate
	· less	· medicate in less amount
	· more	· medicate in e☐essive amount
	· Part of	· medicate only a part of total amount
	· As Well As	· medicate wrongly
	· Reverse	· medicate in a wrong way ☐reverse)
	· Other than	· accompanied with une☐pe☐ed complication

− social background (stress, celebrity, followers)
− misunderstanding of a rule/guideline
− oversight
− simple mistake
− timing has shifted
− economic problem
− problem on information ☐e☐ce☐s, shortage, inaccurate, confusion, a myth, a rumor, and folk remedies)
− character ☐leaving all to others, negligence, stubbornness, overestimation, a person easily elated)
− with a psychiatric disorder
− which noti☐esa falsehood
− with too much suitably
− the in☐uence of eating habits

We analyze human factors for medication risk with HAZOP as shown in Table 4.5.

Table 4.5　HAZOP for human factors in medication

Secondary keywords	HAZOP guidewords	Result	Effect	Frequency	Cause	Safety measure
No/None	Do not medicate					
Less	Medicate in less amount					
More	Medicate in excessive amount					
Part of	Medicate only part of the amount					
As Well As	Medicate wrongly					
Reverse	Medicate in a reverse way					
Other than	accompanied with unexpected complication					

4.3　HAZOP and Rehabilitation for Dysphagia

A) Swallowing phases and risks

In the acute phase of cerebrovascular disease, head injury, and cervical cord damage, it is critical to correspond according to a rapid change of patient condition. Moreover, more efficient rehabilitation should be performed after the acute phase of diseases, and taking nutrition certainly. In the phase of rehabilitation, risk management for swallowing is essential for preventing aspiration pneumonia. Furthermore, in the chronic phase at home or in nursing home, the necessity of securing QOL (quality of life) of a meal is important without overlooking a patient's dangerous sign.

However, as for the contents of the care which surround the patient of each phase, patient care are carried out in the circumstances with crossed variably and various occupational descriptions. Although the bottom of safe swallowing is indispensable, the fact is that many hours cannot be spent in the spot of care for only dysphagia. Care staff and family may be aware of the fear that the maintenance of the patients strongly depend on the correspondence to the problem under dysphagia which has conceived a possibility of exerting danger on a life very everyday. Moreover, even if it is the method of enhancing swallowing function and safety, it cannot be practical if it takes complicated procedure, time, and effort.

In this chapter, the actual condition which aims at more efficient correspondence in dysphagia and the bottom rehabilitation of dysphagia, or the actual scene of care taking advantage of HAZOP is introduced.

B) Pharyngeal Phase
1) Risks in pharyngeal phase

According to Table 3.5, pharyngeal phase are categorized up to the risk rank C and over. At the subnode "laryngeal elevation, airway obstruction" the risk ranking is increase in D and E. Thus, laryngeal elevation and airway obstruction is a climax of safe swallowing, and if this function work insufficiently, the risk of aspiration will increase remarkably. The second highest risk is "epiglottis falls" in a subnode, it seems that we may regard it as a series of movements united with "laryngeal elevation, airway obstruction", since epiglottis falls down on the piriform-fossa side by the larynx carrying out with laryngeal elevation passively, respiratory tract closure takes place as a result.

Next highest risk with much distribution of C ranks, is the phase of closure of nasopharynx by contact with the velum and posterior pharyngeal wall, and this prevents bolus from penetrating to the nasal cavity of food. And this is the phase, "closure of the oral cavity with tight closing of body and base of the tongue, the velum, and hard palate, to prevent backflow into the mouth further".

These functions not only close nasopharyngeal cavity tightly and intercept the nasal cavity and the mouth, but they secure intraoral pressure, and the role to which bolus is made to transport so that negative pressure is produced by the esophagus and the pharynx which result in the flow from oral cavity to esophagus.

Furthermore, bolus passes the upper esophageal sphincter (UES). The esophageal entrance closes by the ceicopharyngeal muscle except the time of bolus passage. When cricopharyngeal muscle loosens to the timing which continues on the elevation of the larynx. In this way, a passage space of the bolus is secured by the elevation of the larynx, and the esophagus entrance opens by relaxation of the cricopharyngeal muscle. Just by line activity of these series progressing duly one by one, one swallowing of the bolus is carried out safely. It is brought about by stagnation of either of these activities that an abnormal condition of a pharynx phase happens. Therefore, the influence for a condition improvement aims at an improvement of condition by performing exact influence to the function which evaluates clearly in the series of swallowing movement.

2) Evaluation of the pharyngeal phase

a) Elevation of the larynx

If swallowing reflex happens, hyoid pulls up and continues to keep the kickback by contraction of suprahyoid-muscles group, the larynx can pull up, epiglottis will fall simultaneously, and the larynx will be closed by contraction of thyrohyoid muscle. Therefore, in order to make larynx closing more reliable, it is required to urge contraction of suprahyoid muscles and a thyrohyoid muscle. In order to make this movement smooth, relaxation of the neck to shoulder muscles and the stretch of the larynx circumference are performed first, when muscles in cervix are in a state of tension. The training is performed according to the situation of the tension of the muscles of the patient in the daytime or before a meal. Furthermore, in voice training, it aims to be useful for preventing aspiration by training the cooperativeness of breathing and utterance aiming at an improvement of larynx regulation and glottal closure.

Training of head elevation given to raising an effect as training to the relaxation insufficiency of superior esophageal sphincter: The Shaker method is validated to incorrect deglutition of the residue, to the laryngeal elevation insufficiency due to the loss of muscle strength of a suprahyoid-muscles group and the pharynx.

b) Strengthen laryngeal closure

Although the larynx at the time of swallowing is closed by fall of epiglottis and the elevation of the larynx as above-mentioned, within the larynx the vocal cord closes simultaneously. When patients have a problem in larynx closing, in order to prevent incorrect swallowing, it is important to strengthen this closing strength. The following training can be mentioned as training which strengthens larynx closing. Adaptation should be chosen for this procedure.

Exercise for vocal cord

This procedure is effective when the risk of aspiration of liquid and saliva is high, followed by pharyngeal residue with insufficiency of the vocal cord closure and nasopharyngeal closure. Movement is performed as a means which strengthens vocal cord closure intentionally. It may be good to use as a method of guiding a cough.

Attentions and contraindications: Patients with hypertension and respiratory diseases should be paid special attention for overload to the cardiopulmonary system, and if the patients have change of vital signs and feeling displeasure, the training should be postponed. It also stops, when condition, like voice gets husky where vocal-cords pathological changes, such as a vocal cord nodule and a polyp.

Supraglottic swallow: swallowing while taking breath and the glottal closure swallowing method

It is the swallowing method which prevents aspiration by removing the residue on vocal cords by expiration immediately after respiratory tract closing before swallowing. In order to swallow turning cautions to breathing, it is supposed that there is an effect which make timing of breathing and swallowing easy to take. It can carry out without using food, a method can be mastered, and actual eating and drinking can also be utilized.

Procedure:

1) Take a light, if possible deep, breathe from a nose and stop breathing. When using food and drink at the same time, as there is a risk of inhaling it together, breath from a nose. When the tracheostomy tube is attached, a tracheal gill hole is closed lightly.
2) Swallow once while stop breathing
3) Breath out "Ha---" immediately after swallowing, or may expirate strongly so that it may cough.

Attention:

1) It is difficult when the patient cannot control feed back movement.
2) If possible, just after breathing you may put food and drink into a mouth. It is good to choose a easy way for the patient.

3) When a swallowing reflex does not occur with saliva, or it already shifts to direct training, you may swallow a little amount of cold water.

4) When carrying out during meal, it is good to carry out for every swallow at each time or for several swallow according to the patients' condition.

c) Soft palate, back wall of pharynx, tongue base

In order to prevent aspiration with the closure of the larynx, the increase of the pressure in the pharynx by closing with the velum, the posterior part of tongue, and the posterior pharyngeal wall and bolus route in the pharynx are important. For those strengthening, adaptation is chosen and the following training is performed.

<u>Movable region expansion training of the tongue base</u>: Tongue movement forward and backward

It is good to perform movement of a tongue using the "resistance movement" which resists the pressure on it when "an active movement (tongue movement forward)" and an active movement are possible. The muscular power of a tongue, especially a posterior part of tongue, is strengthened.

<u>The Mendelson method</u>

It is the method of aiming to maintain at the position which carried out a hyoid and the larynx to elevate at the maximum, to loosen superior esophageal sphincter by raising the pressure of the larynx, and to make residue in the pharynx remove. It shall be effective also as a method of the improvement and extension on a hyoid and laryngeal elevation being obtained and acquiring the effect of decreasing pharynx residues and aspiration also as a compensatory method of swallowing.

Method:

Extract power and return to the state before swallowing, after pointing so that swallowing may be stopped in the place where pharynx contraction reached the peak position of laryngeal elevation, and maintaining several seconds as it is.

Attentions:

1) Because acquisition of this procedure is a little difficult, this maneuver is adapted

for the patients who are able to perform laryngeal elevation and to adapt the feedback movements.
2) As this methods prolong apnea state, patients with coordination disorder with respiration and deglutition should not be adapted.
3) The patients with abnormal muscle tone in the neck and shoulder pay special attention to the application of this methods.
4) Petitions, such as change of the vital signs during the training and feeling displeasure, are cared about.

Head elevation training: Shaker method

It is a method used for the insufficiency of the oricopharyngeal opening in the esophagus entrance part. It shall be effective when the patients shows insufficient elevation of the larynx, residue in the pharynx, and aspiration during swallow caused by weakness of suprahyoid muscles.

Pushing method

Closing strengthening of the velum, a pharynx back wall, and a posterior part of tongue may be obtained as a secondary effect of the following pushing method.

d) Training for insufficient opening of cricopharyngeal muscle

Balloon opening

It is the method of extending opening insufficiency of a cricopharyngeal part using the balloon catheter for urethrae, and improving bolus passage insufficiency. There are several sorts of methods as shown below.

Adaptation:

Although there is cricopharyngeal insufficiency of a entrance of esophagus, there are no views on the inflammation nor ulcer of this part, and patient's physical condition in general should be good. The portion for dilatation can be decided by Videofluorographic Swallowing Study (VFSS), a balloon is actually inserted in the position, and a position suitable for extending is decided. Moreover, before and after inspection, swallowing of liquid or jelly is tried, and the effect is checked instancy.

Method:

There are several kinds of maneuver.

1) Intermittent dilatation: Using a spherical balloon catheter, put a balloon on a narrowed area and repeat contraction.

2) Drawing-out method

-- Swallowing synchronous drawing-out method:

Putting in a catheter to an esophagus, extending a balloon and pulling lightly with saliva swallow

-- The simple drawing-out method:

Using sylindrical balloon to draw out, without synchronizing a swallowing reflex

3) The balloon swallowing method:

Using a spherical balloon catheter, if it inserts to the pharynx, a balloon will be extended, and swallow as it is.

4) Sustained-expansion method:

Fix to the narrowed area checked by swallowing imaging using a cylindrical balloon, and detain for 10 to 20 minutes.

Shaker Method

A supine position is taken, head is carried out on elevation so that the tip toe of a leg may be seen, where both shoulders are made not to float from a floor, and movement which puts power only into suprahyoid-muscles part is performed in order. Attentions and contraindications:

1. It takes care so that strain of muscles other than suprahyoid portion may not be strengthened.
2. Natural breathing is carried out during Shaker method. It warns against straining by force or stopping breathing.
3. There are contraindications when there is a disease of cervical cord. When there are hypertension, cardiac disease, non-exploded aneurysm, adaptation is judged according to the patients' condition.

e) Eating Training

When oral ingestion is possible, aspiration can be prevented or the reciprocal swallowing method is used together even if there is pharynx insufficiency and aspiration is observed. In that case, in accordance with the reciprocal swallowing method, the texture of food, the quantity of a mouthful volume, and a posture of the body and neck is relevant in order to perform safe swallow.

(1) Selection of a food texture

Suitable food texture help mastication, bolus-formation, and movement in the mouth. Although what is called "unit foods" is used because of the restriction of manpower in many cases in supply of food for patients in the hospital, unit food scattered in the mouth of the patients who is difficult to perform bolus formation. In such case repeated food intake cause aspiration and it is not an ideal direct training for deglutition disorders. If possible, food which can easily transfer in the mouth under the insufficient condition of mastication and bolus formation could be used with thick or starchy sauce. In case of pharyngeal dysphagia or insufficient bolus sustain in the oral cavity, we should pay attention to the volume of liquid or moisture in oral cavity.

(2) Posture

When the mobility of tongue or lips is scarce and formation of bolus and the transfer in the mouth are difficult, patients would take the reclining position in bed or wheelchair so that bolus can move according to the gravity. The angle of reclining will be changed according to the condition of bolus transfer in the oral cavity. In the most severe case with dysphagia the upper half of the body being raised from a floor 30 degrees so that bolus move by the gravity. However, when pushing down about 70 degrees or more, the angle of a hip joint will open in the usual reclining wheelchair and the stability will be bad, and the body will come to slip downward, patients should be placed in bed or wheelchair with tilting.

Patients are served for taking food because they can not see the table if the upper half of the body are pushed down. Even in such case patients should keep their head position in a little flexion posture.

It becomes easy to carry out operation which does not need to push down to 30 degrees, and the most suitable position will be decided. In such position patients can see the food on the table and take the food to the mouth.

(3) Food container

In case of pharyngeal disorders the choice of cup for drinking liquid is important. Patients with dysphagia are tend to aspirate with the glasses with an ordinary thin mouth, because they take the position with their cervix prolonged and the bolus move quickly to the pharynx result in aspiration.

We usually use the commercial cup cutting a part of the edge. If the patient can perform straw drinking, a commercial cup with a straw can be used. If the patients can aspirate the liquid carefully, they can adjust volume of the bolus and the timing of swallow result in safety swallowing. If not, patients should be fed by the spoon. Even if the patients aspirate with puree, it is good for liquid ingestion for gelatin jelly to take the tea hardened moderately and a sport drink.

(4) Adjust bolus volume and pace

In the case with difficulty in the pharyngeal phase, bolus volume are needed to adjust for the patients. Some patients have the ingestion custom for large bolus volume and the quick pace of ingestion before the illness. In such case the danger of bolus overflow from pharyngeal space result in aspiration if much quantity is sent to the pharynx. It may be required to urge cautions by speaking suitably, checking notes in notice or respecting the intention of the patients, considering the eating habits from before. Sometimes we should be aware of eating habit of the patients and get the information listening from patients or family, and form a safe bet over many hours.

For adjustment of the amount of mouthfuls, selection of the spoon which is not too large is effective in many cases, and when the patients takes much amount of soups unconsciously, it is good to make a vessel smaller and to urge cautions.

(5) Attention for liquid taking

Since moving speed of liquid in the mouth is quick, flows into the larynx from the pharynx, before swallowing reflex drive, cause coughing and aspiration in many cases. Even when the oral ingestion of the devised food can be carried out, ingestion of liquid may take cautions.

For the patients who tend to aspirate liquid and whose swallowing reflex delayed, puree are used for decreasing the velocity of bolus and guide the bolus safely to esophagus. The degree of thickness of puree are decided by Water Swallow Test (WST) and Repeated Saliva Swallow Test (RSST). The laryngeal movement during swallowing and drink test with thick liquid are also used. If the thickness of the food get too hard beyond necessity, the taste may be spoiled, and care should be taken so that motivation of eating and drinking may not be reduced.

6) Substitution swallow

Think swallow

It is the method to urge to be aware of (or to think of) (bolus swallow) being conscious of the rhythm of digestion or bolus formation. This method is effective for the patients trying to digest without adequate mastication or coughing with liquid.

Spraglottic swallow

This is the method of swallowing with the timeing of breathing. Patients will take the timing of breathing and swallowing intentionally and stop the breath (and close vocal cord) just before swallowing. It is effective for the patients who have aspiration just before or during swallow movements. This maneuver will be effective if patients can inspirate lightly before stop breathing and can expirate deeply after swallow.

Head rotation

When a right and left difference appear in pharyngeal passage, it is effective to rotate the head to the side which is hard to pass before swallowing, and it is more effective to turn head to the bottom a little. This position (front sideways swallowing) make the bolus easy to pass the pharynx. In order to remove pharyngeal residues patients swallow once in the front position and then swallow turning the head to the affected side (after-swallowing sideways swallowing). This is the volume effect of pharyngeal space that turning to the affected side results in increase the space of intact side and bolus can easily pass through the intact side and, prevent aspiration.

Frequent swallow

When the patients cannot swallow the bolus at once and show the sign of wet voice, stimulates two or more swallowing after one swallowing are recommended. Especially this procedure is recommended for the patients with wet voice in order to prevent residues in pharynx. In case of difficulty in saliva swallow small amount of cold water or jerry will be used to initiate swallow movements. In such case alternative swallow of liquid and jerry is used for training (alternative swallow).

Application of the frequency where mutual swallowing and two or more times swallowing will be decided according to the patients condition. When the patients dysphagia is slight, carrying out this procedure to the last of the meal can reduce aspiration and coughing.

The compensatory swallowing method is carrying out ingestion with careful attention to notes, although it will be the requisite for adaptation the patients being able to carry out intentionally, and it can also expect to aim at improvement in the function.

f) Correspondence to meal

(1) Circumstances

It is important for patients with dysphagia to take a meal with attention and concentration to the food for safety. The situations for taking food differ patient by patient, we should be aware of the following points, and transfer the information to the family and care giver.

Environment of mealtime
Be careful to the noise of the circumferences, such as television and a chat, and make atmosphere with the music which the patients can relax with.

Environment of a patient
In a large dining room in a hospital a staff is carrying out the dinner tray under other patients who finished eating previously in the meal, and even if he or she say "Please take your time", the patient will be in a hurry for eating. It is better for the patient to be seated far away from the exit.

Care givers will finish their meal before serving for the patients so as to make the patient hurry for the meal. If the patients is introduction of the rehabilitation or difficult to pay attention to the food, the patients could be served in their individual room.

Environment of communication
Neither the care worker nor the observer carried out the experience of ingestion simultaneously with a patient. As soon as the patient take special food for dysphagia into the mouth, we tend to ask the patient "Is it delicious? How is this meal?" We must keep in mind that the patient will be forced to answer your question and we will ask the patient after checking their swallowing conditions.

Environment of attention
Is there something near for the patients to draw attention? We should keep patients away from putting on a side what diminishes concentration as much as possible. There should be nothing that pulls interest of the patients other than a meal in a side: the newspapers and magazines, telephone rings, sound of television, and a pet going back and forth.

(2) Attention
Consciousness
Level of consciousness is critical especially for the patient just after the acute phase of illness. If awakening time is short or not periodic, it is better to start rehabilitation

according to the timing of good mental status and to enhance mental status.

Is the patient conscious of eating?

It is important for the patients to think themselves of eating and keep the attention to eat such as not coughing or spilling. Special attention should be paid to the patient who have a habit to eat quickly, take large volume of food into their mouth, and difficult to drink liquid.

As the method of cautions, patients should be aware of the way of eating by checking orally or by notes, or by putting the message of notes on a table.

Oral hygiene is also important

A desk message

To understand the patients habit, way of thinking, pride, ability of reflection, and memory is very important, and suitable message should be used. For patients who is sensitive to a written message, devise telling a message with an illustration will be used.

Basically it is important to enjoy eating. We should explain the patient that the message is the caution which prevent the dysphagia patients from pain such as cough and aspiration.

(3) Education for care workers

The guidance about the structure and mechanism of swallowing

First, care workers should be educated for understanding of the mechanism of mastication and deglutition that they are a series of movements and complicated motion. Next, they should understand the patient condition which they take care of.

The most important thing to understand is that the patient with dysphagia can eat with various maneuvers, awareness to swallow and attention to eat, and that the care for dysphagia is indispensable to the patients.

For example, some family do not know that they can observe swallowing movement by checking by the up-and-down motion of the larynx. Thus it is important to let the family and care workers know the overt signs and symptoms for checking a severity of dysphagia.

Instruction of foods for dysphagia
It is ideal that nutritionist perform instruction about the selection method of the swallowing foods according to the ability of deglutition, the point of the device of cooking, the volume of a meal.

Caring for method
When care is required, it teaches about a suitable food texture, a posture, the amount of mouthfuls, and the care method.

4.4 Application to Clinical Pathway

A) Clinical Pathway in health care
1) Clinical Pathway

A Clinical Pathway (CP) was first introduced as critical pathway by Caren Zander, who is a registered nurse of the New England Medical Center, for the management in the patient care in a hospital in the 1980s. In addition, CP is defined as having summarized all the medical examination schedules of the patient under hospitalization, and having made the chart according to the time course. And in order to carry out suitable management efficiently and to draw the greatest effect to patients belonging to the same diagnostic group, each procedure which constitutes the whole medical treatment is set in order, and "critical course" are estimated from the viewpoint of time course to the end point.

First of all, CP is a view generated by the operations research (OR) which developed in the United States. OR is the method of obtaining useful solution and carrying out a simulation to it in military research, planning of production, a transportation problem, using the plan technique using mathematical science and modeling. OR basically developed with the military background in Britain in the 1930s, and the research on OR showed the highest effect in anti-aircraft gun cartridge for saving 20% cost per shoot-down of enemy plane. Henceforth, OR came to draw attention in the United States, and spread in the field of industry or management plan. OR also applied to mathematics such as linear programming, dynamic programming, a multivariate analysis, a waiting line theory, PERT/CPM, and game theory, and it will lead to the analysis which utilized the computer (Figure 4.5).

In addition, OR is used to maximize profits when many product is produced from the same materials or resources and to seek the course completed in shortest time although two or more points must be patrolled. Moreover, there is no restriction in the target category and solution technique, and OR can evaluate on fixed standard from things which can be evaluated not only quantitatively, such as time, distance, and volume, but qualitatively such as the degree of satisfaction and favorable impression. Therefore, OR was suitable to develop CP at the place of the medical area related to various factors related to patients.

Medical standardization and introduction of the fixed amount payment system (DRG/PPS) of the medical expenses by diagnostic group classification started, and the CP actually spread widely as a means to exclude the basis of cost calculation, and the futility of medical expenses in the United States. When CP was introduced to Japan in 1990, it was expected operating efficiency and medical quality, and there were circumstances which began to be earnestly used for the viewpoint of joint care at the beginning. Now medical doctor creates these in the form of hospital treatment plans at the time of patient's hospitalization, and they uses a system which obtains medical treatment fee by using standardization CP, and diagnostic

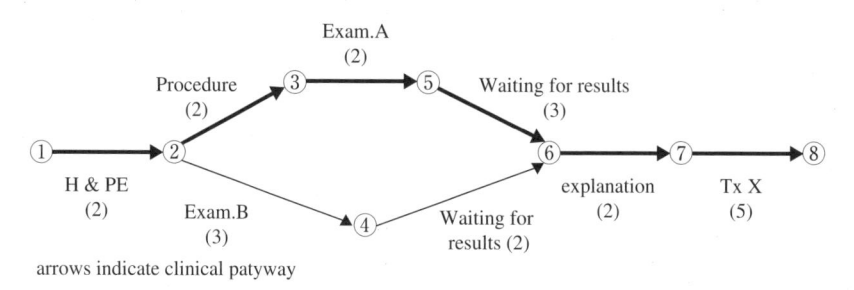

Figure 4.5 PERT and Clinical Pathway

group classification evaluation (Diagnosis Procedure Combination; DPC diagnostic group classification) from 2003. DPC system is introduced into 62 of the advanced treatment hospitals for the purpose for reduction of medical expenses.

2) Preparation to Clinical Pathway

With clarifying a schedule plan and the shortest course of a route in OR, the direction link (combination the starting point and the going direction are clearly shown to be) will be made when work is considered as a link and the starting point and the terminal point of work as nodes. Since the chronological sequence relation of processing between works exists, the time course which connected these links is made. Furthermore, it can be considered that working hours are the dignity to a link. In this way, directed graph with the starting point and the end point is created, and the network graph which gave dignity is called arrow diagram. Arrow diagram makes us possible to find required working hours. The whole time course will be shortened if the longest way from the starting point of an arrow diagram to an ending point can be shortened. The longest way mentioned above is called critical course, and to form the optimal work plan, it is necessary to improve the items on this pathway.

Without omitting the indispensable contents about medical treatment, inspection, or care according to a diagnostic group, CP sets up along with a time-axis, and the whole picture which completes and practices the procedure is indicated to be the contents of the CP. Therefore, if you understand work contents correctly, it becomes possible to advance management so that it may not deviate from the time line along with CP. However, since all the medical staff must be premised on the capability of the performing a task within CP, the quality of a ward or the whole hospital will be reflected indirectly.

3) Making Clinical Pathway

In many cases CP is created based on the knowledge and technology which hospital and professionals have. There are three steps of CP creation. That is, 1) to write out all the contents of treatments and care according to the time course, 2) to create the contents of medical treatment or care introduction using the evidence, 3) to improve CP with analysis of a case which deviates from CP.

Table 4.6 Progress of Clinical Pathway

− The first step −
To write out all the contents of treatments and care according to the time course

− The second step −
It has begun in the stage of standardization of a medical care, and uniformity of a medical care. (though it seems that the effect is still restrictive). Investigation of a patient questionnaire (PS and enforcement analysis (time, contents, cost, and literature consideration (EBM)) are performed. It is reported to leads to shortening of hospital days at this stage. Promotion of team medical treatment and improvement in the quality of a care also begin to progress completely.

− The third step −
Clarification (CQI, increase in efficiency) of the improving point of the whole hospital that an improvement progresses by variance analysis and data practical use (TQM), and promotion of the advantage of the full-scale passing method can be aimed at.

Moreover, even with most sophisticated CP a deviation case arises from the time line, and such deviation is called variance. Variance analysis means to investigate the reason to deviate. It becomes possible by conducting this analysis to get to know the defect of CP and the key of reexamination.

There are two types of variance, positive and negative one. Examples of negative variance are as follows: association of unexpected complications, failure of reservation of examination, delay of the diagnosis, failure of a nurse's inspection/ disposal check, and refuse of patient and family to acceptance for leaving hospital. The important point of these example is a human factor which has a cause medical staff to turn into a practice or factor about the system. First of all, since CP does not regard the human factor as a priority factor, it is reasonable to become such a result. Thus, it is important how this negative variance is decreased especially from the viewpoint of human factors, when we practice CP smoothly. The element which is the target of CP is shown in Table 4.7. Among them aspiration pneumonia caused by swallowing difficulty is very important, because incidence of aspiration pneumonia is highly frequent in elderly people, because the fatal ratio is high, because its medical expense is large, and because it is a disease which leads to extension of hospital days by recurrent pneumonia.

Table 4.7 Objectives and results of Clinical Pathway

＜objectives for clinical pathway＞
・to improve frequency
・to decrease medical cost
・to shorten hospitalization rate
・to standardize treatments of procedures
・to decrease risks for patients
・to promote care coordination
・to standardize deviation
・to promote informed consent
・to promote patient satisfaction
・to promote quality of medicine

About the problem of a system, by using a computer, it has become possible to manage and to prevent from delay of working, and the ever-advancing improvement is aimed at in recent years. Considering that the medical flow from evaluation to treatment of dysphagia and pneumonia is clear from the viewpoint of a specialist, and that fatality ratio among elderly people is high in the developed country, CP specialized to dysphagia or aspiration pneumonia will be needed. One reason for this is that the discretion for examination and treatment of dysphagia is not clear in Japan. Another reason is that CP of pneumonia would have a lot of variance, and that the procedure would be difficult to standardize.

B) Application of HAZOP to Clinical Pathway
1) Significance of HAZOP in Clinical Pathway

Though it is true that team approach for treatment and care of swallowing difficulty are necessary, as a matter of fact there are quite a few hospitals and institutions which have enough professionals both quantity and skills. And since reference on CP does not mention about the influence of the execution capability in an individual or a team, the human factor taken up by HAZOP is left behind.

HAZOP focused in this book is an inquiry system of risk and aims at identifying the hazard of a process, and a problem on operation. It is as above-mentioned that these points may serve as element of variance on CP management. I think that HAZOP can lead to safer and smooth operating management by performing CP creation and management in the style in consideration of the conditions which become a serious risk factor from the contents beforehand analyzed by HAZOP. Moreover, by HAZOP, since it becomes possible to carry out the simulation of the role of each occupational description in a medical team, the result is also brought to the management on performing a task (quality administration). Furthermore, about the medical risk management in connection with the direct management on CP obtained by HAZOP, it can contribute to the production of a system for higher quality medical performance by including in the management manual of CP.

2) HAZOP in Clinical Pathway

Clinical pathway is the timeline with individual procedure with which each medial staff will take responsibility. Basic notion is that medical procedure is one of project managements.

In the clinical (or critical) pathway only when the critical point (milestone) have been achieved, we can move forward to the next step. The critical point contains goals and objectives for medical examination, treatment, rehabilitation, and

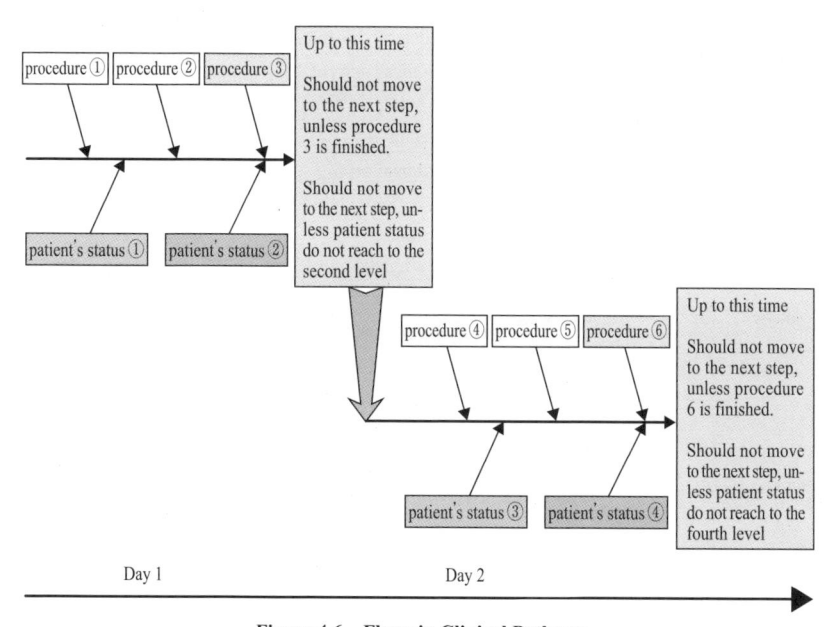

Figure 4.6　Flows in Clinical Pathway

care.(Figure 4.6)

When a deviation occur, and when the goal have not been achieved by the critical point, we must think about how to catch up with the critical point or change goals. If the patients do not meet the criteria for the critical point, medical staff should rethink about the condition of the patients.

This procedure is applied by HAZOP.

3) Clinical Pathway and WBS sheet

The CP contents for dysphagia, which a nurse should do in an acute phase of the cerebral infarction, are shown in Table 4.8. The physical assessment is one of the main items shown in the subwork. From a viewpoint of a human factor, there are two ways for a nurse to check, subjectively they asks a patient about the checking contents, and objectively they carries out various inspection and checks to a patient. In both way they writes down the result in a checklist.

Table 4.8 Acute phase: WBS in physical assessment

Node No.	Person	Main work	Subwork (primary guideword)
Acute phase	Patients (family) & nurse	Physical assessment	· vital sign (4h, if needed)
			· neurological sign (EOM, pupil)
			· visual field
			· lung sound
			· other cranial nerve 　· IX, X: uvula elevation, curtain sign, gag-reflex, oral sensation 　· X, II: tongue movement, tongue atrophy, deviation, fasciculation (1hr, 2 to 4hrs, needed)
			· sputum (character, cough, swallow)
			· saliva (sawallow)
			· voice (dysarthria, horse voice, wet voice)
			· repetitive saliva swallow testing (RSST)
			· bowel sound
			· higher brain function (understanding, judgement, attention, memory)
			· Motor symptoms, DTR, sensory symptoms

4) Correlation of Clinical Pathway to HAZOP

Figure 4.7 is displayed in accordance with the figure of CP of project management, and this figure shows cooperation between sections. It turns out that what is called the display of CP is extremely similar to what showed the work content according to section.

In this case CP consists of training. Since there is enough time in nursing and procedure, other training which needs time becomes critical.

The work content which takes time to a, b, c, d, e, f, g, h, and i, respectively is applied. CP is decided based on the standard hour concerning such procedure. Here, since the flow of the procedure of a, b, and c serves as the longest time, this result is reflected to the CP. However, if procedure in d, e, f and g, h, i is extended long enough compared to the procedure in a, b, and c, deviation will be produced the original flow of the procedure.

Figure 4.8 showed the relation between CP and the extra time of procedure

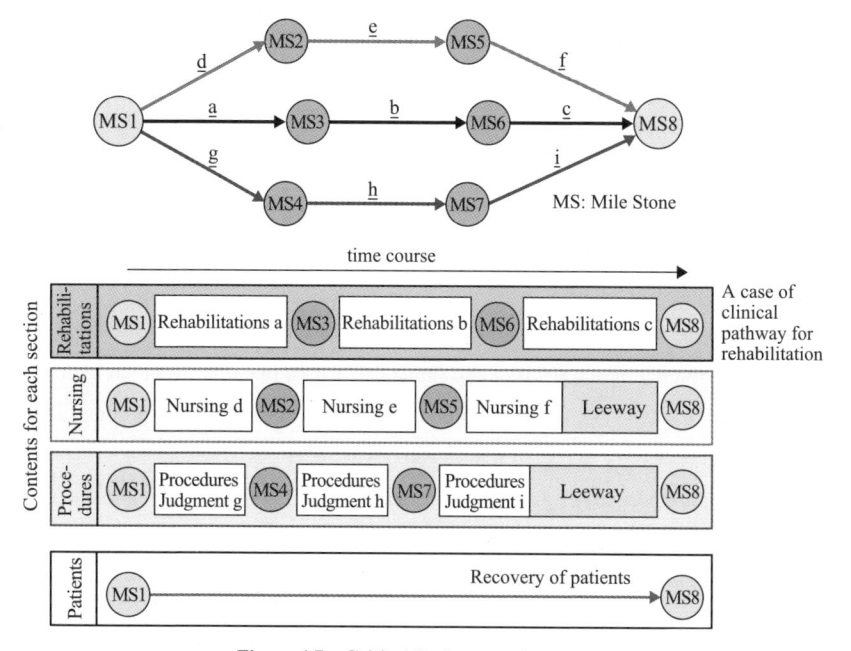

Figure 4.7 Critical Pathway and contents

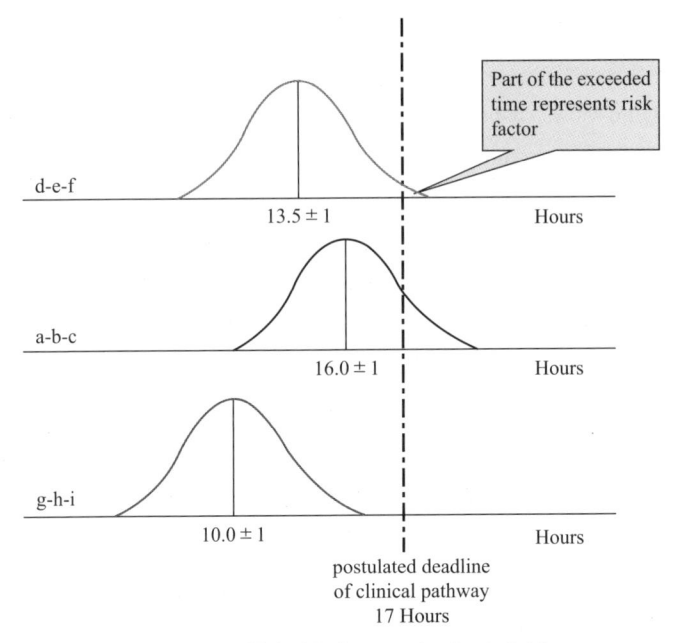

Figure 4.8 Clinical Pathway and estimated risk

assuming that each procedure is carrying out the normal distribution. When the time which d-e-f in a figure assumed at the beginning is extended, the domain which surpassed CP time (here 17 hours) is equivalent to a risk.

Next, we will think about the time exceeded from CP. Figure 4.9 shows working hours according to standard deviation.

As shown in the figure, it turns out that domain B which must extend the original assumption time by about 2 times, and domain C which must be extended by about 4 times exist. Conversely, the domain ended earlier in domain D will produce extra time, it is not necessary to regard it as negative variance.

The standard hour carrying out each procedure is decided from clinical data. 70% of patient is considered to be settled in this standard hour. From the viewpoint of engineering Table 4.9 showed the extent of deviation.

It is estimated that the CP in which 70% of patient can be executed in this standard hour is an accurate one. In this case, it is presumed that about 10% will be carried

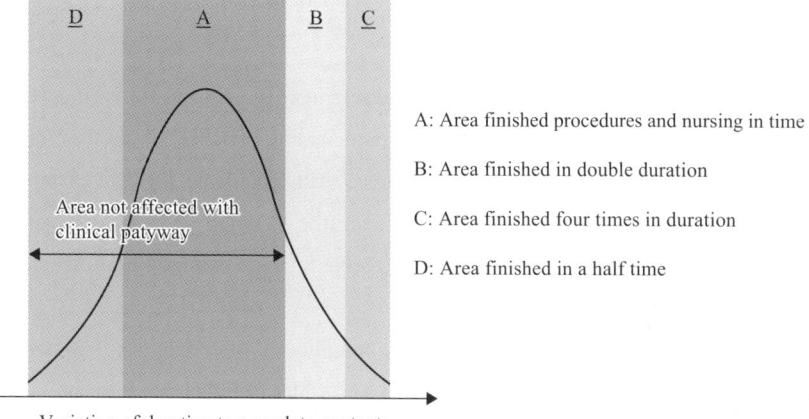

Chapter 4　Application of HAZOP for Risk Management in Dysphagia　*101*

A: Area finished procedures and nursing in time

B: Area finished in double duration

C: Area finished four times in duration

D: Area finished in a half time

Variation of duration to complete contents
Duration for procedures in standard distribution

Figure 4.9　Time course of execution of contens

Table 4.9　Time cource of execution

Time course	Possiblity of complete procedures in time	
	very high accracy in time	high accuracy in time
Area finished in time (A+D)	95%	85%
Area finished in double duration (B)	5%	10%
Area finished in four times in duration (A+D)	0.50%	5%

out within double in time. It is also presumed that about 5% carried out within 4 time longer period. This rate becomes large when assumption accuracy is bad. Since it is presumed statistically that a delay element of this level exists, the scenario which can be considered by using HAZOP is created, and it is an effective method for improvement of the stability and the profit of the management in a hospital.

When carrying out HAZOP of CP, guidewords like Delay, More, As Well As, and Other Than can be considered. Scenario evaluation will be carried out in the case with delay of procedure, the case with extended time, the case with additional variance, and the case with an unexpected event.

5) Clinical Pathway and deviations

The example of deviation of physical assessment in acute phase is important. The point of a problem can be probed for participating member's brainstorming. If participating member are experienced persons, many problems, incident examples, and the tips from experience will be enumerated in detail. When participating member carries out HAZOP, it becomes possible to share common information on medical risks (risk communication).

The treatment and care for dysphagia is complicated with many staffs, medical facilities and systems, and the result varies according to influences intricately and mutually. For this reason, the flow of the procedure among the staff is critical to make CP.

Conclusions

1) When deviation occurs in CP, the influence will be considered and measures will be taken. This pattern of thinking is HAZOP itself.
2) The problem which did not consider the item shown in CP by conducting HAZOP analysis at the beginning may be probed. Moreover, there is also the necessity of transferring the contents drawn by HAZOP analysis to CP.
3) The scenario which can be considered by HAZOP should be created, and it is an effective method for improvement of the stability and the profit of hospital management to consider influence, a measure, and a cause.
4) Reexamination is required when many examples which do not meet a pathway have come out, even if 70 % of the patient meet the critical points at the beginning. Moreover, the stage of CP can be pulled up by introducing accumulated evidence into CP positively.

4.5 Application of HAZOP to In-Home Care

According to the report of Japanese Ministry of Health, Labor and Welfare on the nation's care system for the elderly in 2007, 4,420,000 people (3,610,000 people aged 65 to 74, 660,000 people aged 75 and over) required system's care in "Needing support" and "Needing care" categories. The poor actual condition of care is reported by media almost every day, and at the same time about 130,000 medical-treatment type sickbeds will be abolished in 2011 in addition to the present condition in the state where it was already saturated. The medical-treatment sickbed of medical treatment which is medical insurance application also serves as a plan reduced to 150,000 floors from the 250,000 present floors. This means that the entrance institution which can apply elderly care insurance turns into only special elderly nursing home and a welfare institution for elderly people in 2012 and afterwards. That is, in order to correspond to the aged people requiring care at home who will increase in number in the near further, it is necessary to consider about a medical treatment and care to the people with dysphagia both at home and at nursing-home.

Since being home is a scene of a life, it is hard to say that training environment is ready from the viewpoint of equipment and human resource. When engaged in a patient under such environment, it becomes important to argue if the condition of it is not ready. Moreover, since the evaluation of dysphagia, which cause aspiration pneumonia and directly to death, is difficult from outlook, correspondence has been made difficult until now. However, since research of this field is progressing splendidly in recent years, tools for corresponding to dysphagia patient is getting sophisticated. If such tools can apply to daily life, sufficient correspondence can be taken to the patient with dysphagia in home care.

- medical doctor
- dentist
- nurse
- dental hygienist
- physical therapist
- occupational therapist
- speech pathologist
- nutritionist
- care manager
- carer
- family

Figure 4.10 Team members associated with dysphagia care

A) Tips for organizing care team for dysphagia

Coping with dysphagia we should keep in mind that team approach is foundations. Since meal and nutrition are actions performed every day, even if it can set up as investigation and practice, when it cannot reappear daily, it will become scarce at a meaning. First, the person engaged in the patient and the frequency of intervention should be clarified (Table 4.10). It is important to know whether there is a circumstance to check swallowing and nutrition condition. Videofluorography (VF) and videoendoscope (FEES) are major diagnostic tools for dysphagia (Figure 4.11). They are useful investigating tools not only for diagnosing aspiration but also for checking the type of dysphagia and/or for evaluating swallowing exercise and food texture. Although going to hospital is needed for performing VFSS, it is recommended to check whether there is any medical institution which perform FEES in a clinic, especially performing visiting FEES by doctors. Moreover, in the case of being home, cooperation of family becomes indispensable and, in the case of an institution, cooperation of care workers and common knowledge of information are needed. Thus, it will be necessary to recognize how much family and persons can cooperate.

It is important for a team to perform realistic organization according to the environment which surrounds a patient. Three models to form interprofessional team are postulated: multidisciplinary, interdisciplinary, and transdisciplinary (Figure 4.12). Multidesciplinary and interdisciplinary team are usually performed

Table 4.10 Role for management for deglutition disorder

1. Management of the original diseases and nutritional state	physician
2. Management for dysphagia	care manager
3. Screening for dysphagia	dental hygienist
4. Diagnosis and evaluation of dysphagia	dentist
5. Planning and preparation for suitable meal	family
6. Instruction for manner of and care for eating	dentist
7. Instruction and assessment for training	homecare nurse
8. Establishment of manner and training for eating	family
9. Oral care	family
10.Dental therapy	dentist

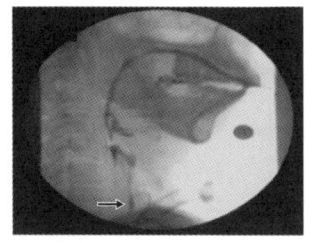

Chapter 4 Application of HAZOP for Risk Management in Dysphagia 105

Videofluorography (VFSS) Videoendoscopy (VESS)

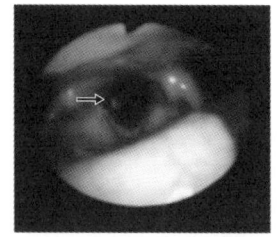

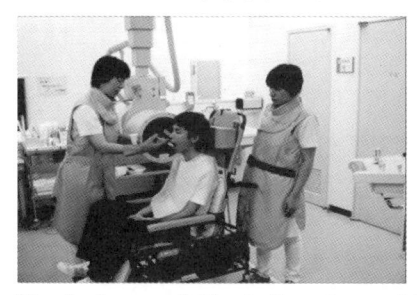

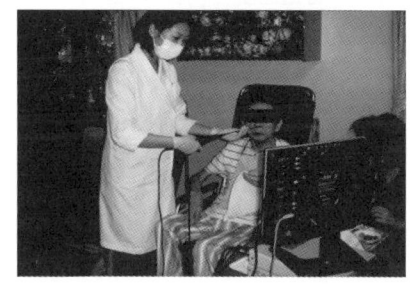

Viseofruolograpyg (left) and videoendoscopy (right). Arrows indicate aspiration

Figure 4.11 Examination of Dysphagia

in a general hospital where it is supposed that each role of medical person is differentiated, and the latter has more interactions between members than the former.

Whereas in trans-disciplinary team, a medical person's role is changed according to a situation to it. As shown in the lower right of Figure 4.12, in the patient of being home, there may be a situation to which neither physical therapist nor a dietitian is concerned with the patient. Under such a situation, other occupational descriptions, for example, a nurse, may have to take charge of a speech therapist or a dietitian role. When it corresponds to a patient with swallowing difficulty with the limited occupational description, it is necessary to learn the knowledge and technology which exceeded the conventional specialty nature if needed, and it may be easy to imagine that it enables to overlap mutual technical field. Especially in-home, the team organization based on the concept as trans-disciplinary is important. Based on the above-mentioned concept, correspondence required for the occupational description engaged in the patient is distributed. If it raises roughly and ten items shown in Table 4.10 can be buried, also in being home or an institution, the

Multi-or Inter-disciplinary Team (ideal team)

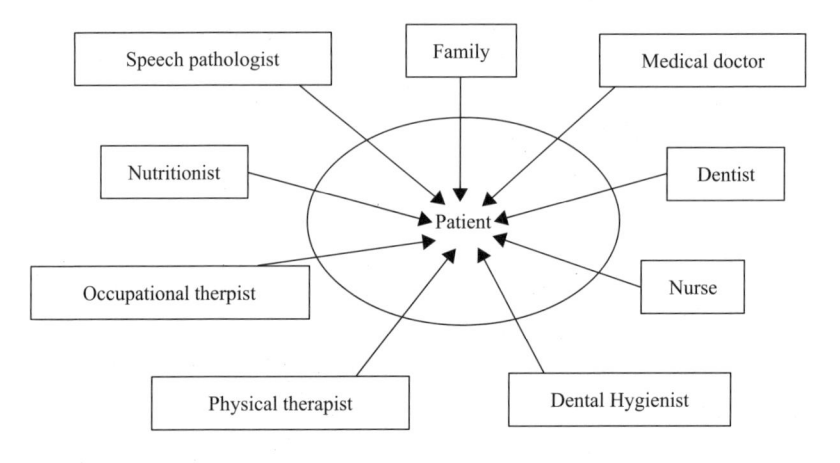

- Speech pathologist
- Family
- Medical doctor
- Nutritionist
- Dentist
- Occupational therpist
- Nurse
- Physical therapist
- Dental Hygienist

→ Patient ←

Transdisciplinary team*

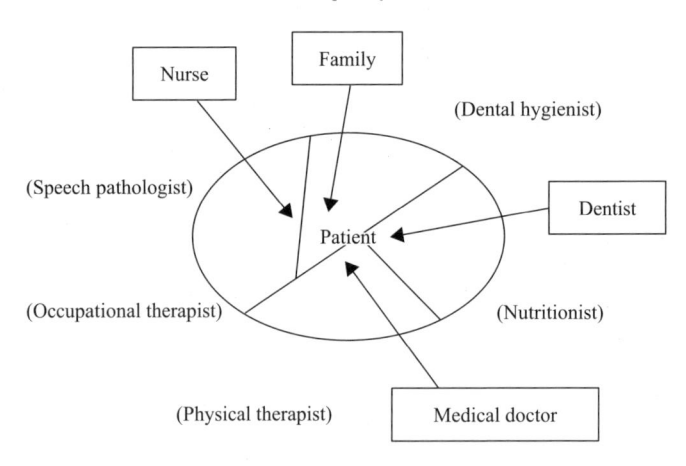

- Nurse
- Family
- (Dental hygienist)
- (Speech pathologist)
- Dentist
- (Occupational therapist)
- (Nutritionist)
- (Physical therapist)
- Medical doctor

→ Patient ←

* Available heath care providers are sharing the role

Figure 4.12 Two types of team approach

correspondence to dysphagia will become possible.

In-home care Table 4.10 shows the example of the role assignment corresponding to a patient. Of course, this is one example and is not always having to be such a team.

B) Case presentation

The patient was a 69 years-old woman and the eldest among three sisters. She had two episodes of aspiration pneumonia after subarachnoid hemorrage, and she postponed eating and fed by pericutaneous endoscopic gastrostomy (PEG) followed by any episode of pneumonia after that. We (dentistry) had a request for investigating swallowing function from the care manager because there is a strong hope for oral ingestion from a family. We informed to the family doctor that swallowing functional test will be performed and if necessary training for deglutition will be started.

The first swallowing examination was performed eight-month after subarachnoid hemorrage. The consciousness level was clear, and the condition of oral cavity is fair though there were several caries. The problem was not found in articulation, utterance, neck movement, and expectoration. The oral hygienist performed a screening test of dysphagia: RSST (Repetitive Saliva Swallowing Test) and MWST (revised water drinker test: Modified Water Swallowing Test) which resulted in normal. Subsequently, when FEES was performed with the posture of 60 degree reclining. The patient were able to swallow jelly, rice porridge, or banana without any abnormal findings. She was also able to digest banana. However, since ingestion had hardly been carried out from taking orally for about eight months, we recommend the family to practice safely and to eat little by little only using all the rice porridge.

Since the frequency we can visit was about once per month, we inform to the family how to carry out rehabilitation training for swallowing. At the same time we asked home-visit nurse to check whether the family carry out the procedure precisely. Although the short-term target was improving training environment including a family, the long-term goal was taken as establishment of oral ingestion,

Table 4.11 WBS of training for dysphagia based on the first examination

Main work	Person	Subwork	Problems and Incident cases	Tips for Work
Training for dysphagia	Trainers (Family)	Check and prepare before training	Fever Sputum Posture at training Food for training	Stop training with fever Stop training with wet voice remains Start at 60 degree Start with porridge
		Training	A mouthful volume Compensation methods Check after training	Tee spoon Check wet voice after swallow Wet voice (expectoration or suction)
	Estimator of training (home care nurse)	Assessment of training	Fever Respiratory state Observance to training contents	Stop training with fever Stop training if prblem Inform to a physician Check and correct the way of training Inform to the dentist if the training unsuitable

since the prominent obstacle was not found. Training based on the result at the time of the first medical examination and evaluation of the situation were performed as shown in Table 4.11.

Since the condition of oral cavity was good, an oral care performed continuously by the family, and several caries were treated in the initial stage by home-visit dentistry. After one week home-visit nurse reported that training using rice porridge can be achieved without any problem, and we decided to start rice porridge only at lunch. (Figure 4.13). After that training by the family and evaluation of a training situation by the home-visit nurse continued, and ingestion frequency and meal texture was made to be hard gradually. Three months later, ingestion of staple food was attained completely. Since the situation of oral ingestion was good, two more months after consulting with a family doctor, PEG was removed, and she had no deglutition problem until now.

This is a typical case who can take in 3-meal staple food from PEG. There are two important factors for the success for training at home. One point is that FEES has been offered at home. Since thorough examination will not be done unless dysphagia is not prominent, in other words, some patients are forbidden to eat because they

Chapter 4   Application of HAZOP for Risk Management in Dysphagia   *109*

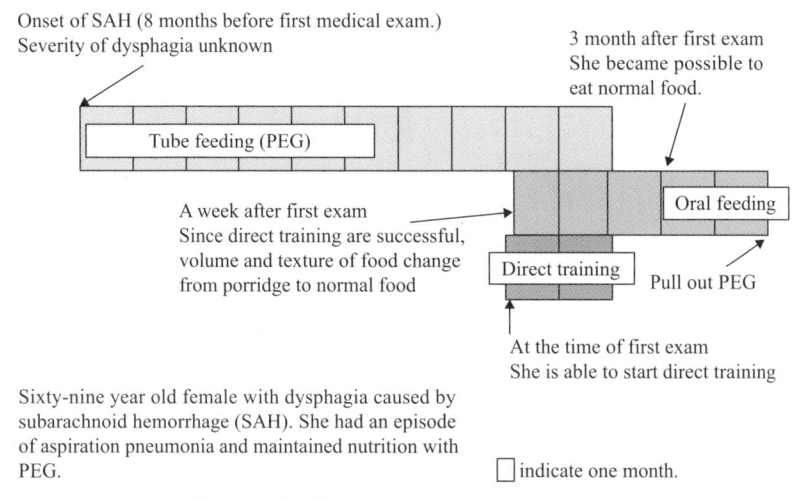

Onset of SAH (8 months before first medical exam.)
Severity of dysphagia unknown

3 month after first exam
She became possible to eat normal food.

Tube feeding (PEG)

A week after first exam
Since direct training are successful, volume and texture of food change from porridge to normal food

Oral feeding

Direct training

Pull out PEG

At the time of first exam
She is able to start direct training

Sixty-nine year old female with dysphagia caused by subarachnoid hemorrhage (SAH). She had an episode of aspiration pneumonia and maintained nutrition with PEG.

☐ indicate one month.

Figure 4.13   Timeline of the patient with dysphagia

do not receive a proper examination. In that sense, a proper examination at the beginning of home-care are very important for the patients suffered from dysphagia. The improvement of examination environment led to a success in this case.

The other key factor is at the point which was able to carry out the role assignment of an actual training person in charge, and also the evaluator of a training situation were well arranged. The family were very cooperative for daily exercise, and collaboration of the family, and a home-visit nurse is considered to have led to the increase in efficiency of training. The important instructions of the rehabilitation training to the family was not only the contents of training but also discontinuous conditions. In addition, the contents of training have continued safely by having been advanced without raising a family's burden extremely as a range which can be performed daily in addition to the visit nurse having checked the training situation.

When we cope with a patient with swallowing difficulty, it is important to secure first the human resource which can diagnose the state of swallowing ability, and the person (for a family to also contain) who meets a patient daily (Table 4.12). Moreover, in order to perform more effective patient care, it is necessary to arrange other occupational descriptions flexibly according to a patient's training environment

110

Table 4.12 Tips for team care

-There must be a staff who can diagnose of the situation of dysphagia
↓ If impossible
When a deglutition condition is getting werse, A patients can be assessed by visiting nurse
-There must be a person who can observe all day
↓ If impossible
It is very hard to take care

or the situation of an local area.

Summary

1) In order to correspond to the patients with dysphagia, especially in-home care, it is important to perform flexible team organization according to a patient's environment or the situation of an local area. The key factors for success are environment of suitable examination, maintenance of the training environment by appropriate role assignment, and instruction of the clear contents of training and a stop standard is important for continuation of training.

4.6 Application to Basic Research for Dysphagia

A) Application to basic research for dysphagia

Swallowing movement are complicated operation not only with the involuntary movement controlling in the brain stem, but the element of a voluntary action with which cerebral function involves (Figure 4.14, 4.15). In this book, HAZOP is used as the risk management tool for complicated swallowing movement. Each process of swallowing movement is taken apart into WBS as Node and Subnode (shown in Chapter 3) (Table 4.13, 4.14) before analyzing with HAZOP. Then, deviations from each process are considered comprehensively by guidewords. In this process unanticipated deviations come appear, and they could be a new clue for development in dysphagia research. In this chapter, application of HAZOP to the field of brain

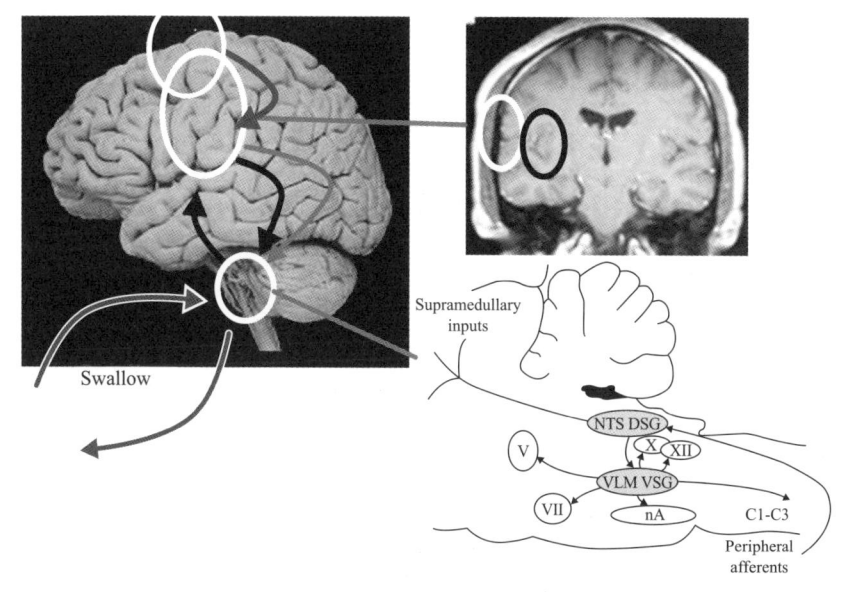

Figure 4.14 Cerebral control of swallowing movement

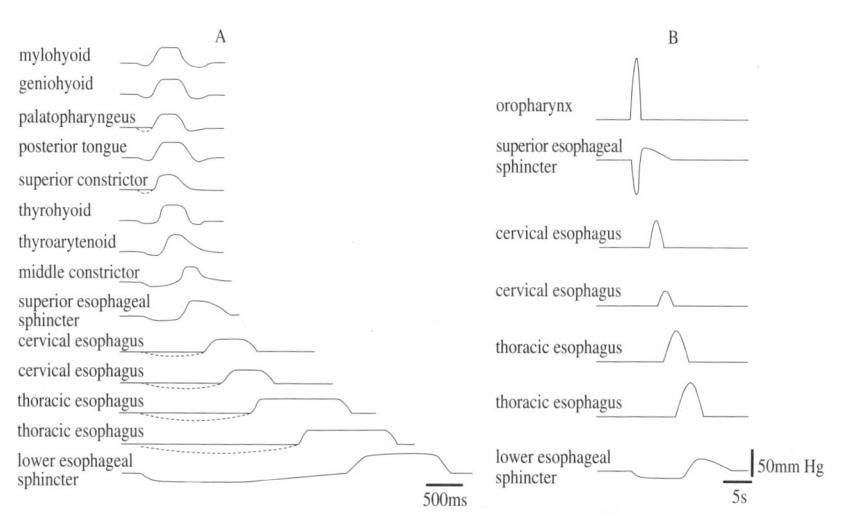

Figure 4.15 Sequential movement of deglutition
(Jean A. Physiological Rev. 2001.)

Table 4.13 Node ingestion and bolus formation

Function	Component									
	teeth	lips	tongue	cheek	maxilla	madible	soft palate	hard palate	salivary gland	posterior pharyngeal wall	lateral pharyngeal wall
Ingest Food	◎	◎	○	○	○	○					
Preserve food in oral cavity											
Prevent flow forward (lips)	◎	◎	◎	○	○	○		○			
Prevent flow backward (oral canal)			◎	○	○		◎	○			
Prepare texture											
cut and grinde	◎	○	◎	◎	○	○	○	○	○		
mix with saliva	◎	○	◎	◎	○	○	○	○	◎		
Form bolus					○						
form bolus with tongue	○	○	◎	○	◎	○	◎	◎	○		
form bolus with plalate			◎	○	○	○	◎	○	○		
Transfer bolus (through oral canal)	○	○	◎	○	◎	○	○	◎	○		
Prevent reflux to nasal cavity (closure of nasopharynx)			○				◎			◎	◎

Chapter 4 Application of HAZOP for Risk Management in Dysphagia *113*

Function		Sensory system						Cranial nerves						CPU		
		taste	smell	thermal	pain	tactile	pressure	V	VII	IX	X	XI	X	medulla	basal ganglia	cortex
Ingest Food		◎	◎	◎	◎	○	○	◎	◎	○		○	○	◎	◎	◎
Preserve food in oral cavity																
Prevent flow forward (lips)		◎	◎	◎	◎	○	○		◎	○	○	○	○	◎	◎	◎
Prevent flow backward (oral canal)		◎	◎	◎	◎	○	○		◎	○	◎	◎	◎	◎	◎	◎
Prepare texture																
cut and grinde		○	○	○	○	◎	◎	◎	○	○	○	◎	◎	◎	◎	◎
mix with saliva		○	○	○	○	◎	◎	◎	○	○	○	◎	◎	◎	◎	◎
Form bolus																
form bolus with tongue		○	○	○	○	◎	◎	○	○	○	○	◎	◎	◎	◎	◎
form bolus with plalate		○	○	○	○	◎	◎	○	○	○	◎	◎	◎	◎	◎	◎
Transfer bolus (through oral canal)				○	○	◎	◎		○	◎	◎	◎	◎	◎	◎	◎
Prevent reflux to nasal cavity (closure of nasopharynx)				○	○	◎	◎				◎	◎	◎	◎	◎	◎

Table 4.14 Node from closure of nasopharynx to cough reflex

Function	teeth	lips	tongue	cheek	maxilla	madible	soft palate	hard palate	salivary gland	posterior pharyngeal wall	lateral pharyngeal wall	palatal arch	supra-hyoid mauscle	infra-thyroid muscle
Prevention of reflux to nasopharynx (nasopharyngeal closure)			○				◎			◎		◎		
Transfer bolus (pharyngeal phase)			◎				○	◎	○	◎		◎	◎	◎
Movement of tongue base														
Clear residue														
epiglottal wall			◎				◎		○	◎		◎	◎	○
pyriform sinus							◎		○	◎		◎	◎	◎
pharyngeal wall							◎		○	◎		◎	◎	◎
Prevent aspiration														
reverse of epiglottis			◎										◎	○
closure of vocal cord														
apnea during swallow														
Transfer through UES									○				◎	◎
Cough reflex														

Chapter 4 Application of HAZOP for Risk Management in Dysphagia 115

Function	Component					Sensory system					Cranial nerves					CPU		
	epiglottis	Vestibule of larynx	pseudo vocal cord	cvocal code	middle pharynx	UES	taste	smell	thermal	pain	tactile	pressure	V	VII	IX	X	XI	XII	medulla	basal ganglia	cortex
Prevention of reflux to nasopharynx (nasopharyngeal closure)	◎																		◎	◎	◎
Transfer bolus (pharyngeal phase)		◎	◎	◎	◎				○	○	○				◎	◎		◎	◎	◎	◎
Movement of tongue base					◎					○	○	○			◎				◎	◎	◎
Clear residue						○															
epiglottal wall	◎				◎				○	○	○	○			◎	◎	◎	◎	◎	◎	◎
pyriform sinus					◎	◎			○	○	○	○				◎	◎		◎	◎	◎
pharyngeal wall					◎	◎			○	○	○	○				◎					
Prevent aspiration																					
reverse of epiglottis	◎								○	○	○	○			◎	◎	◎		◎	◎	◎
closure of vocal cord		◎	○	◎											○	◎			◎	◎	◎
apnea during swallow						◎									○	◎			◎	◎	○
Transfer through UES					○	◎			○	○	○	○			○	◎			◎	◎	
Cough reflex																					

mapping research for dysphagia are introduced.

B) Research on swallowing control

Although the cause "damage in cerebrum" appears frequently in the HAZOP table in Chapter 3, the mechanism of central swallowing control has not been clarified. By making a HAZOP sheet which is introduced in this book, a working hypothesis can be made, that the participation of cerebral cortex to the swallowing center in the medulla oblongata. Since voluntary control (intentional control) can be performed in swallowing movement, the process that supplementary motor area → motor area → medulla oblongata center could exist. If we take this process apart into WBS, nodes can indicate as follows.

1) Input of motor initiation from supplementary motor area to primary motor area
2) Input from primary motor area to medulla (NTS DSG) via pyramidal tract
3) Input from NTS DSG to VLM VSG in medulla
4) Input from VLM VSG to nucleus IX, X

Deviations of the first node listed above by using guidewords are shown in Table 4.15. The region prior to primary motor area including supplementary motor area is considered to have the memory impression in the past, like other association cortex such as somatosensory cortex, visual cortex, and auditory cortex. It is assumed that the motor activity experienced before is stored in the region in premotor area (motor engram). Therefore, since motor engram memorized here will disappear if the damage of the region in premotor area occurs, the skillful movement is suffered. From the HAZOP table, the signal form supplementary motor area to motor area could result in either a condition of decrease or increase of the signal (or fall of control). Although not yet clearly solved as a cause, the deviation with question mark is assumed from a mechanism by HAZOP. Thus, a new research question becomes clear by conducting HAZOP analysis. Here, we introduce about the problem of the cerebral control mechanism of swallowing movement extracted from the above-mentioned process.

Table 4.15 Gvideword and deviation

Secondary guidewords	Deviation	Effect 1	Cause · Cause of deviation · Root cause
None/No	No input from SMA to primary motor area	No volitional swallow	Cerebral infarctin (bilateral?, unilateral?) Brain injury (bilateral?, unilateral?) Brain tumor
As Well As	Extra input from SMA to primary motor area	Dificulty in initiation swallowing	Cerebral infarctin (bilateral?, unilateral?) Brain injury (bilateral?, unilateral?) Brain tumor Parkinson disease?
Delay	Delay of input from SMA to primary motor area	Delay of timing of swallowing	Cerebral infarctin (bilateral?, unilateral?) Brain injury (bilateral?, unilateral?) Brain tumor Parkinson disease?

Although many researches are reported on brain mapping study in swallowing with fMRI, MEG, PET, the cortical mechanism of swallowing has not been clearly understood. When studying by brain mapping, we find it difficult that swallowing movement are greatly influenced by person's posture and is restricted in compared to the real deglutition movement by motion artifacts of face and head. Recently there are reports of the functional brain mapping using near-infrared spectroscopy (NIRS). NIRS can measure hemoglobin concentration using the dispersion light of noninvasive near-infrared light, and can mainly detect change of the blood flow in the cerebral cortex (Figure 4.16). The apparatus of NIRS is relatively small and mobile, and it is the feature for swallowing research to keep free from posture in a seating position. We are studying on brain mapping about various types of swallowing by NIRS, which we can take the same posture as everyday swallowing movement.

The probe covered on the primary sensorimoter area of the face, mouth, and pharynx. The band fixation on a jaw was not used because it would produce motion artifacts. The person maintained in the seating position and carried out tasks for swallowing movement. Each timing of swallowing movement was determined using the simultaneous record by the interface for video photography systems.

118

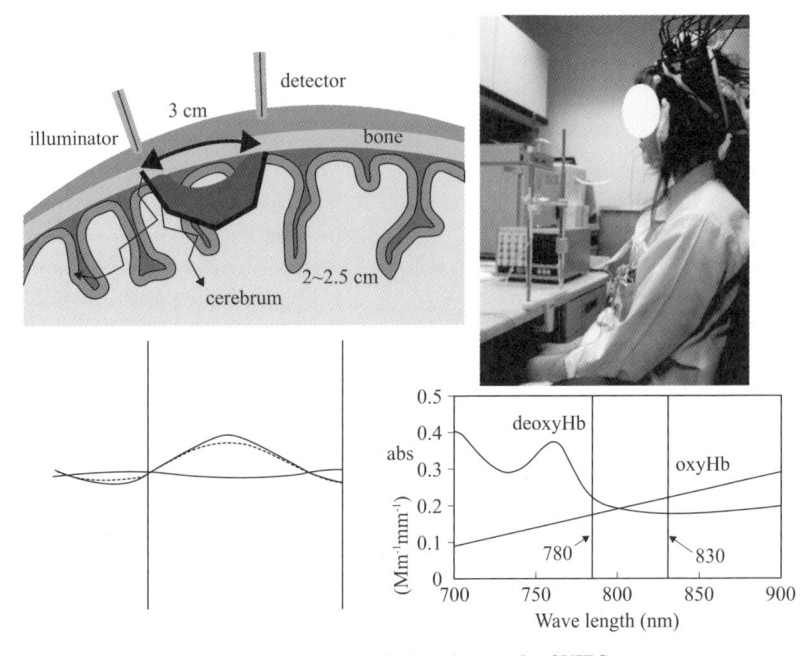

Figure 4.16 Theoretical backgrounds of NIRS

For investigating continuous movement, the blocked task of mastication, pursing, tongue movement, or continuous saliva swallow was performed for 10 second for 10 times. Furthermore, we studies on single trial for swallowing movement. Command swallowing movement were summated for 20 times on the basis of the time of a swallowing reflex start. For non-command swallowing movement, extension tube were fixed so that an tip might come to 4cm from a row of teeth, and distilled water was dripped in with the infusion pump in □ ml□sc, and the time of a swallowing reflex being automatically started for a person naturally. Although the amount of bolus by which a swallowing reflex is initiated are different individually and it was 4 to 20ml, and the amount of bolus was almost constant in the same person. About swallowing movement, summation was performed 20 times to analy□ed.□igiti□er e□uipment was used for the position of the probe immediately after measurement, position information was ac□uired, and the picture was expressed as software in □□ mapping.

Chapter 4 Application of HAZOP for Risk Management in Dysphagia 119

The questionnaire on the condition for experiment was performed to each person, and there was not restriction during swallowing movement by wearing of equipment. Analysis of blocked trial at the time of digestion, an orbicular muscle of mouth, a tongue, and swallowing movement showed the pattern with which NIRS signal distribution differs, respectively. (Figure 4.17) Figure 4.18 showed totalHb, and deoxyHb change in command swallow. The signal pattern of the oxyHb rise and the deoxyHb fall was broadly seen considering the sensorimotor area of cerebrum. The pattern of the signal strength of oxyHb of command swallow is different to that of non-command swallow. On the other hand at the time of non-command swallowing movement, the brain functional activities of this part were falling. In the comparison at the time of non-command swallowing movement and command swallowing movement, the NIRS signal was extensively changed largely in the latter (Figure 4.19). Moreover, in large digestion movement cause motion artifacts, and the NIRS signal oxyHb, totalHb, and deoxyHb affected showed the pattern of the fall or the rise altogether.

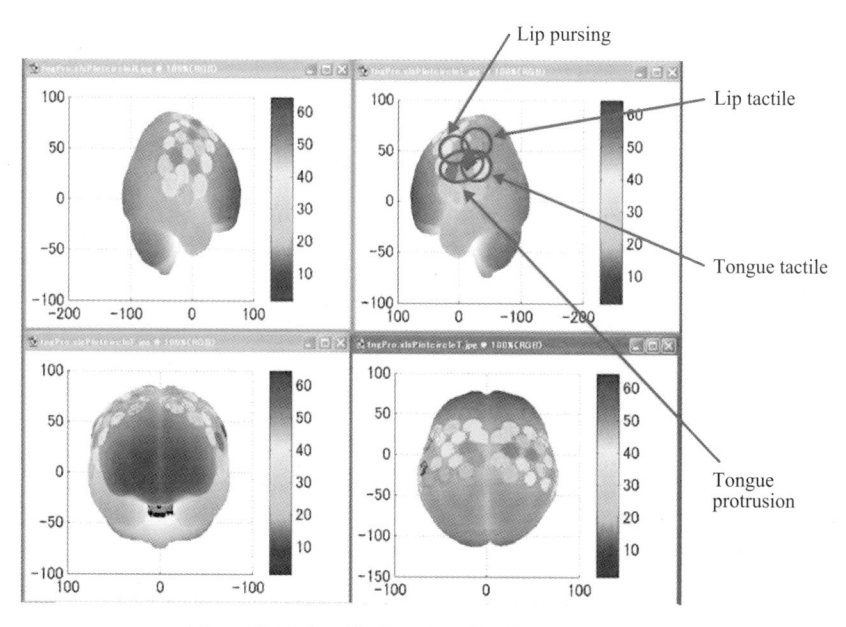

Figure 4.17   Localizafion of swallowing component

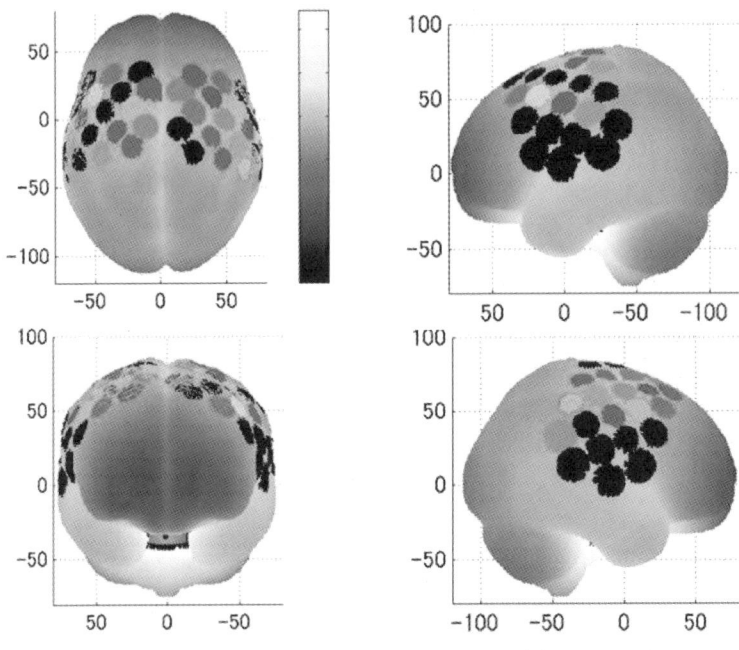

Figure 4.18 Command Swallow (n=25)

In this examination, the point that brain activity is widely activated by command swallow compared to non-command swallow, and the point that right side was more activated than left side, and it is in accordance to previous reports of fMRI in a supine position. Moreover, since the signal of different spatial pattern was seen in tongue protrusion, oris contraction, and pharyngeal contraction. Thus, the activated portion relevant to each movement could be separated. Although NIRS can detect signals in surface of the brain, it is necessary to combine brain function data from MEP or MRI.

Furthermore, a possibility that command swallowing (≒ voluntary swallowing) was controlled by a different mechanism from non-command swallowing (≒ natural swallowing) was suggested. It is important how cerebrum involves in the initiation of swallowing movement because patients with dysphagia feel difficult to start swallowing, and their swallow movement often results in volitional type.

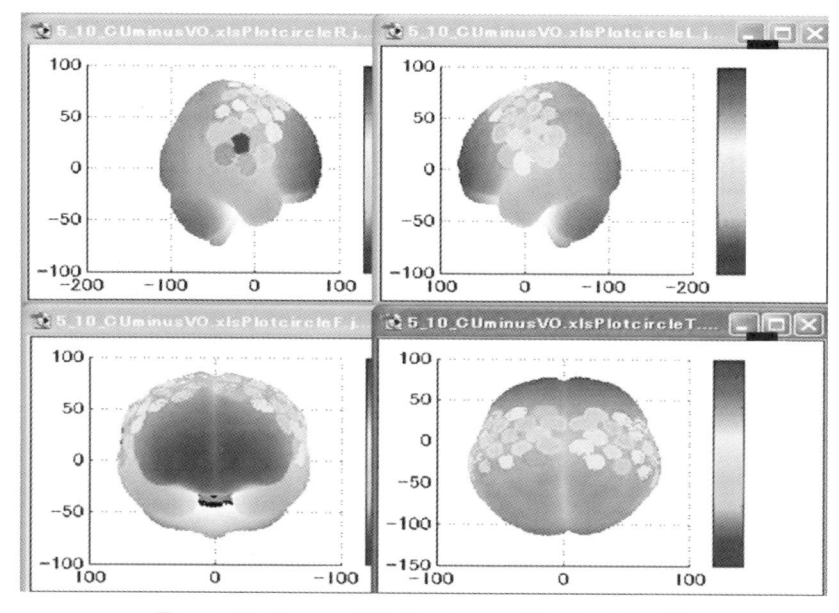

Figure 4.19   Command VS. Non-command (subtracted n=25)

This phenomenon shed the light to the rehabilitation of swallowing difficulty. When considering measures especially in HAZOP, command swallowing becomes difficult in patients with dysphagia, and to take procedures to induce swallowing movement (like thermal-tactile stimulation) is efficient for this type of patients. Originally HAZOP is an approach used for general risk management and risk assessment. In addition, HAZOP is performed to analyze a phenomenon comprehensively in the process of WBS, and its application to basic research and clinical study is also possible.

Summary

1) HAZP is a powerful tool to find and analyze research questions with comprehensive analysis.
2) Central mechanism of swallowing movement is under investigation by using HAZOP.

■ Editor

Masanaga Yamawaki, MD, Ph D, MMA
Associate Professor, Department of Neurology
Tokyo Medical & Dental University

Tohru Nomura, MA
Department of Professional Development
Tokyo Medical & Dental University

■ Authers

Chapter 1. Masanaga Yamawaki, MD, Ph D, MMA
Associate Professor, Department of Neurology
Tokyo Medical & Dental University

Chapter 2. Tohru Nomura, Ph D
Department of Professional Development
Tokyo Medical & Dental University

Chapter 3. Masanaga Yamawaki, MD, Ph D, MMA
Associate Professor, Department of Neurology
Tokyo Medical & Dental University

Chapter 4
4.1 Atsushi Okawa, MD, Ph D
Associate Professor, Department of Orthopedics
Tokyo Medical & Dental University

4.2 Tohru Nomura, Ph D
Department of Professional Development
Tokyo Medical & Dental University

4.3 Mitsuko Shimizu, SLP
Department of Rehabilitation, Saitama Rehabiritation Center

4.4 Yumi Chiba, Ph D
Associate Professor, School of Nursing
Chiba Prefectural University of Health Sciences

4.5 Haruka Tohara, DDS, Ph D
Associate Professor, Department of Dysphagia Rehabilitation
Nihon University School of Dentistry

4.6 Masanaga Yamawaki, MD, Ph D, MMA
Associate Professor, Department of Neurology
Tokyo Medical & Dental University

■編著者紹介

山脇正永　（やまわき　まさなが）

 1988 年　東京医科歯科大学卒業、国保旭中央病院研修医
 1990 年　東京医科歯科大学神経内科勤務
 1992 年　バージニア州立大学医学部生化学教室研究員
 1996 年　東京医科歯科大学大学院医学研究科博士課程修了（神経内科学）
     埼玉県総合リハビリテーションセンター医員
 2000 年　東京医科歯科大学医学部講師（神経内科）
 2003 年　東京医科歯科大学医学部准教授（臨床教育研修センター）
 現在に至る
  医学博士、医療管理政策学修士
  日本内科学会総合内科専門医、日本神経内科専門医
  日本摂食・嚥下リハビリテーション学会認定士

野村　徹　（のむら　とおる）

 1977 年　大阪大学大学院修士課程修了（専門領域：構造物の破壊）
 1977 年　日本製鋼所（株）室蘭研究所勤務
 1986 年　日本鉱業（株）主席技師長・審議役
 2001 年　マーシュジャパン（株）バイスプレジデント
 2009 年　テクノ・スタッフ（株）コンサルティング・グループ・マネージャー
 現在に至る
  大阪大学大学院客員教授・非常勤講師
  東京医科歯科大学大学院非常勤講師

Risk Management for Dysphagia: Application of Hazard & Operability Study (HAZOP)

2010 年 2 月 27 日　初版第 1 刷発行

■編 著 者────山脇正永・野村　徹
■発 行 者────佐藤　守
■発 行 所────株式会社 **大学教育出版**
    〒700-0953　岡山市南区西市 855-4
    電話（086）244-1268　FAX（086）246-0294
■印刷製本────サンコー印刷㈱

© Masanaga Yamawaki, Tohru Nomura 2010, Printed in Japan
検印省略　　　落丁・乱丁本はお取り替えいたします。
無断で本書の一部または全部を複写・複製することは禁じられています。
ISBN978-4-88730-974-6